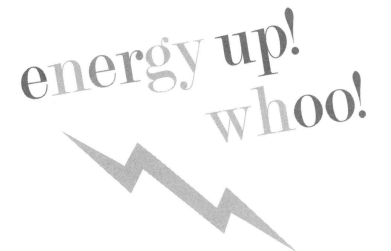

energy up!

energy up! whoo!

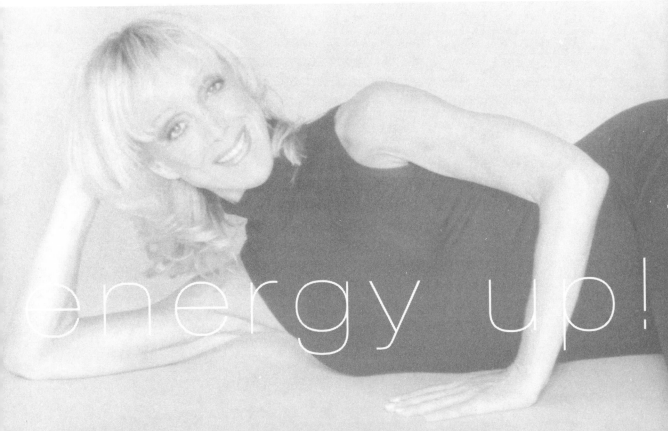

energy up!

energy UP!

Shed Pounds, Get Fit, Gain Stamina, and Turn on Your Power with This Unique Program

high voltage

G. P. Putnam's Sons
New York

G. P. Putnam's Sons

Publishers Since 1838

a member of

Penguin Putnam Inc.

200 Madison Avenue

New York, NY 10016

Library of Congress Cataloging-in-Publication Data

High Voltage.

   Energy up! : shed pounds, get fit, gain stamina, and turn on your power with this unique program / by High Voltage.

       p.   cm.

   ISBN 0-399-14311-4

   1. Weight loss.   2. Reducing diets.

   3. Reducing exercises.   4. Nutrition.   5. Physical fitness.   I. Title.

   RM222.2.H45   1998

   613'.7—dc21   97-34831   CIP

Printed in the United States of America

10   9   8   7   6   5   4   3   2

This book is printed on acid-free paper. ∞

BOOK DESIGN BY DEBORAH KERNER

Illustrations © Charles Björklund; interior photos by Roberto Ligresti; makeup and hair by Kevin Shapiro for Zoli Illusions.

Take a Stand,

Join the

Cosmic Command—

And Yell—

Energy Up!

Well, my name is **High Voltage** *and I'm here to say*

If you want to get with it, you'll do it **MY** *way.*

I'm an **energy conductor** *with a futuristic vision.*

I arrived from Planet Volta in a cosmic collision!

I'm here to save the world from a lack of en-er-gy.

We're going from the New Age to the Voltage Dy-nas-ty.

Take a Stand,

Join the Cosmic Command—

And Yell—Energy Up!

My magic's done with glitter, of that there is no doubt.

You've got **to glitter on the inside, to glitter on the out.**

I'll get you in **shape,** *and you will feel*

What it really is like, to have **flex appeal!**

Take a Stand,

Join the Cosmic Command—

And Yell—Energy Up!

Take a Stand,

Join the Cosmic Command—

And Yell—Energy Up!

1984,
© Jeffrey Gurian
and Betsy Berg;
produced by
Kurtis Blow

TO MY FAMILY

To my adorable mother, Tona—I know it has never been easy being my mother (and it's not gonna get much easier after you read this book!). But thank you for never giving up on me. I love you very much. To my precious father, whom I call Poppo— thanks for supporting Mom through the nightmare I put you both through. I love *you* very much too. And to my darling little sister, Bonnie, whom I adore with all my heart, and who learned exactly what *not* to do, by watching me; and her talented husband, John O'Gallagher, who has (kind of) expanded my musical tastes (it's so cool to have a jazz genius in the family). The tide has turned—and a new game has begun.

TO GABRIELLA RICH

I still hear your wonderful voice and exuberant laugh in my head; you left us much too soon. You will always be in my heart, now and forever. Your energy will always be a part of me. I love you . . . and miss you very much.

ENERGY UP! WHOO!

Contents

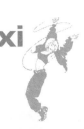

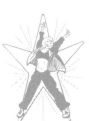

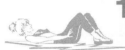
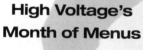
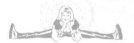

energy up!

Introduction

My motto is **"ENERGY UP! WHOO!"** I shout it—loud and clear—every time I meet someone, every time I walk into a room, every time I answer the phone. (It sometimes makes the walls shake.) To me, "Energy Up! Whoo!" is my wake-up call. Like a mantra—but a loud one!—it centers me, empowers me, and energizes me (and others) **BIG-TIME!** In my opinion, we've already gone from the Stone Age to the Ice Age to the New Age. Well, my little cutie pies, welcome to the **VOLT**-Age, the age of energy!

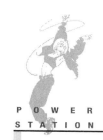

Stop Dieting! Live Fit the High Voltage Way!

If you've gone on diets and weight-loss plans before, and maybe lost a few pounds only to see them come right back, then I bet you're skeptical about my program. What can I possibly tell you that you haven't heard before, right?

Well, hear me out: If you're ready to accept **a new, energy-charged way of thinking that will change your relationship with food forever,** and will result in your *staying motivated, living healthier, and feeling more energetic every day,* then stick with me and let me help you transform your life.

But in order to lose weight permanently, to get fit *and stay that way,* you have to be motivated to accept a whole new, permanent way of life. It's a completely new ball game! Forget anything you've read or heard about diets. I'm in charge now.

Sweetie, you have to be ready to **LISTEN** to what I tell you (and I'm warning you—some things are **NONNEGOTIABLE!**). I'll tell you just what I tell my personal clients—the models, actors, TV stars, and entertainers, and some of the country's top, fitness-conscious executives, who not only pay me handsomely for my services, but get results.

You have to be willing to play follow-the-leader—and
I'M THE F@#!*ING LEADER.

AND YOU WILL WANT TO FOLLOW. I know because I've seen it happen. Usually it's slow at first. But once you experience the **HIGH VOLTAGE HIGH**—once your body starts changing and your energy starts flowing—**IT'S LIKE MAGIC, PEOPLE!** My clients get up in the morning; they put on music; they dance around; they act in ways they've never acted before. And they're being told by someone who looks like a cross between Tinker Bell and something out of an action comic book **THAT THEY CAN DO ANYTHING THEY WANT IN THE TWINKLE OF AN EYE.**

I WANT YOU TO TAKE CHARGE OF YOUR LIFE—not just what you eat. Because how you eat, why you eat, and what you eat says a lot about how you feel about yourself.

Come on . . . when you feel good about yourself—when you CARE about yourself—you don't treat your body like a garbage can! But when you get to the point where you love yourself—and your life—you will *naturally* eat what is good for you, **WITHOUT HAVING TO THINK ABOUT IT.** Anybody can do it. (*I'm* living proof of that, as you'll see in the chapter ahead!)

Just as you can train yourself to run a marathon, you can train yourself to enjoy healthy, nutritious **LIVING** foods like fruits, vegetables, grains, and organic meats, instead of the latest "heart attack on a plate" from the Golden Arches (which, in my opinion, should be standing over a cemetery!). When you consider that McDonald's feeds ten percent of the American public—**IT IS FRIGHTENING!** And McDonald's is certainly not alone—how about Burger King, Wendy's, Pizza Hut, Taco Bell, and the rest of those guys? No wonder there's a virtual obesity epidemic going on.

My job is to turn you off that lifestyle and food-style, to the point where you can do—or eat—*anything* you want. The key is that you'll want different things. (Trust me: I live this way because I want to, not because I have to.) Besides, what are you giving up? Food that clogs your arteries, drugs you up, and makes you fat? The only thing you're going to gain is energy; the only thing you're going to lose is weight.

In the course of my program, you are going to change what you **LIKE** to eat. You are going to replace old food patterns with new ones. If salty snack foods

POWER STATION

THE KEY TO CHANGE IS IN YOUR BRAIN. THE REST IS SURE TO FOLLOW!

are your downfall, when three-thirty P.M. rolls around and your internal clock says it's snack time, you're going to *automatically* reach for a crunchy red apple or a bunch of juicy grapes, instead of that handful of potato chips—*not because you're exercising your willpower, not because I tell you to, not because you know it's "good" for you, but because* **YOU WANT TO.**

I have been talking about the same way of eating for a long time. When you eat the Voltage way, you:

- **Eat no flour, no sugar, no salt.**
- **Eat as close to nature as possible.**
- **Avoid processed foods.**
- **Drink water—lots of it.**
- **Stay away from those new, nonfat snacks (which are loaded with sugar!).**

It sounds tough, but what's so hard to understand? **EARTH TO PEOPLE! THIS ISN'T RADICAL!** It's just common sense (which, unfortunately, isn't so common anymore).

Do you *really* think you can lose weight (and stay healthy!) on a diet that includes sugary cookies, no-fat (but high-calorie) cakes, and even ice cream? Do you really think that high-protein diets (you know the ones I mean!) that have you loading up on artery-clogging bacon and eggs, cheeseburgers and steaks, are going to serve you well *in the long term?* Come on . . . who's kidding whom?

The problem is, common sense gets tossed out the window when the latest fad shortcut to weight loss comes along.

The Great Information Binge

FACE IT: Every day the "experts" tout a new diet breakthrough, a sure-fire cure-all, a guaranteed-not-to-fail, thirty-day wonder diet. I think, Puh-leeze, spare me, every time I read about another diet "breakthrough," and wonder how long it'll take—*this time*—for *the other experts* to start tearing it down.

In case no one remembers anymore, **in order to lose weight,** *you still have to keep the number of calories you eat lower than the number you burn.*
Body chemistry doesn't change!

It's **MIND-BOGGLING** that anyone can keep their head on straight with all the information (and misinformation!) that's out there. We've spent so much time worrying about proper proportions, correct food combinations, fat grams, calories, more carbs than proteins (or is it the other way around—this month?) that our brains have become obese on information alone!

Now, I don't claim to have invented any of this, by any means. The knowledge is out there. Sift through all the diet hype and bullshit and you'll find others telling you a lot of the same things that I will. Many of you are listening too. But not enough. *Not enough people are tuning in and taking action!*

I say it's time to go on a **MIND DIET!** *I am as concerned about flabby thoughts as I am about flabby thighs!*

That's where I come in. Other messengers haven't been able to attract your attention—even though there are some powerful fitness-oriented personalities out there. But I'm a cosmic cheerleader!—moving at a hundred miles an hour! I'm hard to ignore!

Why Americans Are So F@#!*ing Fat

Before we start working together, it's important to understand why obesity has reached such epidemic proportions. What's happening? I'll tell you: We're moving less . . . and eating more, that's what. Portion size has gone **OUT OF CONTROL!** *Gargantuan* restaurant servings have thrown us all off course. And a serving size is a joke. Take the cereal most people eat for breakfast every morning. The recommended serving size for most cereals is about 3/4 cup. With 1/2 cup of skim milk, that's about 180 calories.

Not so bad, right? **BUT THAT'S NOT WHAT'S HAPPENING.** Most people are eating at least **TWICE** that amount—for a hefty 360-calorie morning meal!

As a result, despite all the books touting the latest diet fad, despite all the exercise videos selling like greasy little hotcakes, despite all those "wonderful" new fat-free foods, the National Center for Health Statistics reports that one out of three Americans over the age of twenty (and more than half of us past fifty!) are now overweight! That's up a whopping twenty-five percent—and accelerating at a rapid rate: eight percent in the last decade, three percent in the last three years alone! Do you know that means thirty-two percent of all men, thirty-seven percent of all women, and even fourteen percent of our kids are overweight! What the hell is going on?

A health and energy crisis—that's what! So, sign on with me and take a cosmic ride away from obesity and straight back into health, energy, and fun. But remember, what I say goes. No excuses, no exceptions.

One last thing. I use a lot of profanity. It's my way of getting your attention and driving home my point. I've found it can get people to sit up and take notice of what I'm saying. If it bothers you, ignore it, but don't let it get in the way of hearing my message.

ENERGY UP! WHOO!

I'M LIVING PROOF THAT ANY *BODY* CAN GET THEIR ACT TOGETHER— IF I CAN, YOU CAN

When people look at me today, they see an exuberant blond dynamo with the body of Barbie and the inspiration and motivational abilities of Norman Vincent Peale. I'm fifty years old and have more energy than a lot of twenty-year-olds. Have I always been like this? No way, sweetie!

What was I like "before" I became High Voltage? For one thing, I knew about addictions firsthand: food, cigarettes, drugs, alcohol, you name it. As an ex-smoker, ex–heroin addict, ex-anorexic *and* bulimic, recovering alcoholic, confirmed food addict, locked-up, onetime totally screwed-up person—who seriously attempted suicide—I think I was put on this planet to be a living, breathing example that any body can get their act together no matter what they've done to themselves.

Here's my story. . . . I'm *certainly* not bragging—but I'm not *apologizing* either. This is all in the past. Now, I'm looking to the future!

My Life BV (Before Voltage)

- My first sexual experience was date rape—at age fifteen, by a neighborhood boy I met at a party.

- At sixteen, I was a featured dancer on the national TV show *Upbeat,* performing with stars like Bobby Sherman, Simon and Garfunkel, and The Lovin' Spoonful.

- Just before I turned eighteen, I left home for California to hang out with all my music people in Laurel Canyon in Los Angeles, then the music mecca of the rock industry. (I'm also talking drugs **BIG-TIME** here, people!) Soon I was pregnant by a soon-to-be-famous songwriter who went on to write some incredibly big hits. I stopped taking drugs the minute I knew I was pregnant (at least I had that much sense!), but I danced up until my eighth month. At the time, I believed it was impossible to raise a child alone, so I gave up my baby boy for adoption. The day I got out of the hospital, I shot heroin in one arm and speed in the other—and I basically didn't stop till I was thirty years old!

∿ **Volt-Note!** ∿

Not long ago, when an Indian guru (reading my aura, no less!) said he sensed an unrelieved hole of sadness in my heart, I knew immediately what it was. I like to think that perhaps, through this book, I'll be able to find my son.

- At age nineteen, I moved to New York and again fell in with a heavy drug crowd. Of course, it *was* the late sixties—so that wasn't hard to do! Soon, I was making front-page headlines in the *New York Daily News,* the *New York Post,* and the *New York Times,* in connection with the drug-related death—and highly unusual "burial" (in a trunk, tossed under the Brooklyn Bridge!)—of a friend.

- Between the ages of twenty and twenty-four, I was partying with Keith Moon, Jimi Hendrix, Eric Burdon, and other rock stars of the era. Back in the late sixties, everybody slept with everybody, so, to be perfectly frank, I was waking up with strangers all the time! This behavior was always alcohol- or drug-related, since indiscriminate sex really wasn't my nature *at all.* I subsequently lost six of my best friends to drug-related deaths and murder, including my live-in boyfriend of five years. Those friends are six of the many reasons I'm so AGAINST AGAINST AGAINST drugs and alcohol today.

- But back then, kids all across the country were drinking and drugging. We were searching for a higher consciousness, and many of us thought that with drugs we had discovered a shortcut to enlightenment. I don't think we realized what we were doing, or that we were hurting ourselves—killing ourselves—until people literally started dropping dead! The love and euphoria we thought we found turned into a nightmare.

- At the age of twenty-five, I married a multimillionaire real estate tycoon and entered the glamorous worlds of transatlantic travel, horse racing at Saratoga, glittering gambling casinos, and luxurious spas. To be brutally honest, it was not a love match, but more of a "business" deal—but we both knew the score. I guess you could have called me a married mistress! My job was to look good and be "fabulous," and I was happy—no, *thrilled*—to oblige.

- My husband was tremendously overweight and I worried about his health. I soon convinced him to go to Durham, North Carolina, to sign up for what's been called "the Rolls-Royce" of weight control programs—the renowned Duke University Diet and Fitness Center, birthplace of the now famous Rice Diet—the whole premise of which was built around removing salt from the diet. Little did I know then that "no salt" would one day be a cornerstone of my own program! I spent four months at Duke to be with my husband (flying back to New York every weekend for my manicures and pedicures, of course!). And while I was there, I learned a lot about healthy eating, diet, and exercise. As for my husband, he lost ninety pounds and got a hair transplant and new clothes—I guess you could say he was my first makeover.

- Inevitably, though, the fast-track life took over. I think of our lives together as a Harold Robbins novel! His money allowed us to travel—we were constantly jetting off to casinos around the world. There were round-the-clock parties. I was doing drugs, booze—and the money flowed. He never complained about my spending his money on anything—and I mean anything—I wanted. I like to say I wore only ten carats and up (God, I was a spoiled little monster!). At one point, I was spending $7,000 a week on clothes alone! Not to mention how much money was going up my nose!

- Eventually, my husband and I made a deal. While he traveled to buy race-horses, I could go to any spa I chose. Needless to say, I was always going to spas—in California, Florida, and London—which is how I learned so much about the business. Besides, since I drank and did drugs, I always needed a place to dry out (this was before I was "upgraded" to hospitals). A lot of people back then used spas as dry-out centers, as well as places to work out, hang out, relax, and be glamorous.

- Spas were fun, but I soon discovered bulimia—bingeing and purging—as a way to stay thin. There was no name for this terrible condition back then; I had no clue that it was even an illness. In fact, I thought I had made a brilliant discovery! Soon I was on intimate terms with the bathrooms of New York City's most glamorous restaurants.

- Finally, at twenty-eight, after years of a flamboyant, drug-and-alcohol-ridden lifestyle (which included mingling with everyone from Arab princes to Mafia chieftains), it all became too much. I attempted suicide by taking sixty sleeping pills, forty Valium, and a whopping vial of morphine in the bathroom of a Madison Avenue coffee shop.

  Of course, even if I was going to die, I wanted to look good (I used to joke that I was the best-dressed drug addict in town!), so before I tried to kill myself, I made sure I was well turned out in a beautiful, little gray Chanel suit, Ferragamo shoes, and a Gucci handbag (but no ID inside).

- I woke up at Bellevue, strapped down and with tubes up my nose! Quickly, my husband whisked me to one of the country's most exclusive dry-out centers, Silver Hill, in New Canaan, Connecticut. There, cleaned up (for the time being, at least), I hung out with celebrities ranging from a society philanthropist to a famous rock musician (to whom I loaned my room for trysts with a fellow patient). Needless to say, he didn't last there long!

- Sadly, my own rehabilitation didn't last long either. Less than a year after drying out at Silver Hill, I was in New York's Mount Sinai Hospital's psychiatric lockup ward, where I stayed for *four months*! This time, the rehab took (this was no country club with doctors, where they served high tea wearing white gloves). Released, I retreated to the Harbour Island Spa, a run-down little hotel spa on the New Jersey shore to take stock of my life— or what was left of it.

- At the Harbour Island Spa, I met Jean Kaufman, a longtime guest and the mother of disc jockey legend Murray the K. Jean was also a pop songwriter of some note: remember the novelty hit "Splish-Splash, I Was Taking a Bath"? Well, Jean took me under her wing; with my own family miles away, back in the Midwest (where my wonderful—and forgiving—parents still live today), Jean became like a second mother to me, nurturing me, loving me for who I really was (and for the first time, I was starting to know who I was too!). In fact, it was Jean who gave me my new name when she bought me a fourteen-karat gold fingernail with a diamond-chip lightning bolt and told me I was her little high-voltage baby!

- Then, while I was getting better and feeling healthier, something extraordinary happened. I experienced what I know some people might call a spiritual rebirth—although those aren't the kinds of words I use. I always say I'm a born-again something—I just don't know what. . . . I knew I couldn't continue the way I had been living, or more accurately, dying.

- Drug-and-alcohol-free for the first time in my adult life, I broke from my husband and the lifestyle that was destroying me. I even gave up smoking cigarettes—I just lit one up one day and got sick as a dog. It was because of some sort of chemical change in my body, and I haven't smoked since (I really wish I knew what happened, so I could share it with all you smokers out there!).

- For the first time EVER, my life was consciously joyful. Plus, working out every day at the spa to loud, fast, heart-thumping disco music, I got high on *endorphins*—the chemicals your body releases naturally when you work out. I felt them kick in just like the drugs used to! Except exercise was a "drug" that was totally safe—and healthy!

● Most important of all, I became self-sustaining—economically as well as spiritually. For some reason, I never thought I could take care of myself and not depend on a man to support me. But the very thing I feared most—*working*—saved me.

Although I entered Harbour Island Spa as a guest, I ultimately became its most innovative director. Before me, they had two uninspiring exercise classes. I designed a new program! This was a phenomenal change for me. For the first time in my life, I had a job. I was earning my own money and I even got my own apartment! I paid the rent myself and decorated it on my own. I put in things that I liked—mirrors on the walls, lots of them (a recurring theme for me, as you'll see!), big potted trees, clean white carpeting, and a series of five-pointed star mirrors mounted on the wall going up the stairs (the first glimmer of my five-point Star Power Plan). When I woke, I experienced feelings of peace and contentment that I never had before. I thanked God for everything. I couldn't wait to go to sleep every night, so I could wake up the next day.

My new apartment overlooked the ocean. Every day, my morning started with a brisk "energy" walk along the boardwalk.

How can I describe my life at Harbour Island? Well, I interacted with literally thousands of guests—greeting them at mealtimes, talking over their problems, leading energy classes. And as I became the true driving spirit of the place, I found myself putting my own experiences to work for me.

I always say I graduated from the University of the Streets—with a Ph.D. in **common sense!**

For instance, it was easy to figure out why most people didn't stick with the typical exercise routines that were popular then. Exercise was so dull no one wanted to do it. Remember, this was the late 1970s—and the fitness industry was still in its infancy. The only fitness star was Jack LaLanne. Jane Fonda hadn't even made her first video!

I became a pioneer. A maverick. I decided to bring what I loved best (and missed) about the nightclub and disco world into the spa—the music, the dancing, the outrageous energy (not the drugs and alcohol!)—to exercise. I installed a disco sound system in the spa's gym. I came up with exercise routines to songs by Donna Summer and Gloria Gaynor ("If They Could See Me Now" was a favorite).

Keep in mind, this was *years* before the aerobics craze. In fact, the term "aerobic dance" was so new that it hadn't even reached the spa world yet. Even so, when the few people who *had* heard of aerobics came to my high-voltage boogie class, and wanted to know about taking their pulses (common practice in aerobics classes to this day), I said, "Don't you dare, darlings. You'll have a heart attack when you see how hard your heart is pumping!" (Obviously, I've always been a wise guy!)

I brought nightlife action and excitement to exercise. And people got excited—in fact, my workouts became a sensation! My boogie class even attracted an audience like a Broadway show. In short order, a high-energy lightning bolt became my logo!

My Life AV (After Voltage)

- By 1981, three years after taking over the spa, I was basking in the amazing success of my ideas. Ecstatic guests told me, "You've changed my

> **Volt-Note!**
>
> At that time, there were no cool exercise clothes around, so I made my own, cutting up old designer evening dresses, putting them over leotards and tights. Plus feathers. Glitter. Boas. Sequins. And it worked. Soon, I was written up in all the local papers. My first big headline, "Spa Star Takes Over Hotel," was light-years away from "Hip Pair Held in Trunk Death."

life." Now *that* was a real high! I started offering a cellulite cream-and-wrap treatment at the hotel, which made a fortune (we called the room where guests got the treatment the Cellulite Retreat!). I even asked my little sister to come in and run it for me (understand, I was building my new life here). And yes, I knew that the treatment results were temporary—*as did my guests*. But when you're going to a certain black-tie affair, or have to look great because you're going to sleep with someone for the first time (or whatever!), nobody cares that it's temporary as long as they see a difference!

- After three years, I don't think anybody could have been happier than I was, or feeling more complete and satisfied. I had finally gained control of my life, my health, my shape. It was more than good—it was ecstasy!

- Suddenly, in a single horrifying day, my world collapsed. After an abrupt change in the spa's ownership I was told in no uncertain terms to "get my pictures off the wall, and get out!"—along with everyone else. The people who took me in were out!—and new owners were on the way. I lost my work, my friends, my business, my home, and even my beloved mentor, Jean Kaufman, who died of heart failure (she was eighty-nine) the very afternoon I heard the news.

- To this day, there is no way that I can describe the emotional devastation I felt. The spa had been my whole world; the people there were my family. Leaving was harder for me than any of the other losses I'd been through. I had already become known there as "the Queen of Energy"—so I was literally dethroned! I fled—back to the Big Apple. Once again, I had to create a new life.

- I have to admit that for a time, I felt lost. There was no one to whom I could explain what I was feeling. But I knew that little spark of voltage wasn't dead yet—and I snapped out of it. It was not long after I returned to New York that I went in for my first round of plastic surgery, something I freely—and joyfully!—admit (after all, I *had* lived a somewhat dissolute life!). Physical aging was something I had never thought about before, and gravity was starting to take its toll. As I always say, if it starts to move, put it back!

- So I went for a total repackaging. Eyes, nose, face, neck, lots of tightening here and there. And collagen lips. I even changed my hair color. Twice. My goal, in fact, was the Jessica Rabbit look. I didn't want to look well rested, I wanted to look supercharged: *Vroom!* A few years later, I did my boobs too, with great results!—or so I've been told! I should have done them long ago!

- Foreseeing the aerobics and fitness boom, I burst onto the New York City nightclub scene as High Voltage, the city's hypercharged, electrifying, cosmic Queen of Energy, back in the nightclub world I used to know. I staged "energy concerts"—and people went wild. I was out to rebuild my empire—little did I know that in New York, it would take a whole lot longer than it had in a sleepy little town on the New Jersey shore!

- I started wearing lots of glitter. Looking back and knowing how psychologically numb I felt from the loss of the spa—and my spa family—I have to admit it was almost like donning armor to keep people at bay. But it worked. My white paper jumpsuits were sliced by silver lightning bolts; glittery, sparkly "cosmic dust" raced from my cheeks to my hairline! I looked like I belonged on the cover of *Vogue*—but on Mars!

- Promoting the joy of "exertainment"—that's exercise plus entertainment (I guess I have always coined my own words)—I threw myself into making working out outrageous and fun, and people, from models to moguls, responded. Everybody was talking about that blond maniac running around yelling "Energy Up!" and getting people to kick off their shoes, stretch, and do push-ups right on the dance floor. My makeup artists painted lightning bolts on people's faces (it was called getting "Volted by Voltage"!). Even then, I never looked on myself as an exercise person. I was something else: an energizer!

   (To be perfectly honest, it usually took a few minutes for people to get used to my looks—and my sound—but once you did, you were hooked! As Eileen Ford, one of my first private clients and the founder of the Ford Model Agency, said in a TV interview on *PM Magazine*, "It's not what she does, but how she does it. She is indeed full of energy. It's an electric thing that transfers itself somehow.")

   Not long afterwards, the *Daily News* crowned me "the new Queen of Energy" (although they never mentioned who the old one was!).

Kicking the Diet Habit

When I was at the Harbour Island Spa, working on a daily basis with men and women who had spent their lifetimes trying to get their eating habits under control—food junkies, you could call them—I quickly saw that while diets sometimes work for the short term, ultimately they are **DOOMED TO FAILURE.** No matter what the diets were—lettuce diets, water diets, grapefruit diets, juicing, food combining—they didn't work. If you've tried any of these over the years, as I have (and I've done them all!), you know what I mean. Three to six months after that kind of dieting, and people are fatter and more desperate and depressed than when they started. It's no co-incidence that the first three letters of "diet" are *d-i-e!* But if diets don't work, what does?

As an addictive personality myself (talk about understatement!), I began to recognize that certain foods, for certain people, are not only energy-depleting, but actually *addictive*—f@#!*ing lethal triggers to compulsive overeating. Working with guest after guest (and testing my theories on myself), I discovered the triggers. *Doughy* bagels and breads. *Sugary* cakes and cookies. *Salty* potato chips.

Lethal Substances: Flour, Sugar, and Salt

Flour, sugar, and salt—three white powders that are as addictive for some of us as those other white powders—heroin, speed, and cocaine—are for others. Given my history, I should have known it!

Let me explain. Although doctors and scientists are reluctant to acknowledge it, **eating certain foods sets off a craving for more of that same type of food.**

If you have toast or a bagel for breakfast at home, by the time you get to the office, are you eyeing the snack cart with Danishes, sweet rolls, and other treats with flour in them? Same thing with sugar: If you munch one cookie, do you reach for another? **HEY, HOW DO YOU THINK NABISCO OR KEEBLER OR PEPPERIDGE FARM STAY IN BUSINESS, ANYWAY?**

As far as pretzels, potato chips, corn chips, and other salty snacks are concerned—they said it themselves: **DAMN STRAIGHT "BET YOU CAN'T EAT JUST ONE!"** It's one of the only times that advertising isn't lying to you!

Now, chances are you may not be conscious of this eating pattern—yet. But that's what I'm here for: to help you **WAKE UP** and make that connection. Hellooo!—**EARTH TO PEOPLE!** It took me a long time to wake up and get conscious. In fact, I was **ASLEEP** at the wheel for the first thirty-one years of my life! Don't make the same mistake I did.

These principles became the building blocks of my new life. Once I lived in sand castles; now I wanted to build a real one . . . not all at once, but with a strong, solid foundation, brick by brick by brick.

So, the first thing you need to know about my program is: No flour, no sugar, no salt—**NO KIDDING!**

Forget About Willpower and Love Yourself

This way of eating has allowed me to stay in shape for more than twenty years (believe it—I'm fifty years old!), with an energy level twenty-year-olds envy, without ever feeling tired or hungry or deprived. Let me repeat: I don't diet. You won't have to either. I also don't have a corner on the market on willpower.

Learning to eat and live this way has *nothing* to do with having willpower. As an addictive personality, I probably have even less natural willpower than you do! The difference is that I've learned to steer clear of ALL the "white powders" that trigger my addictions.

In the course of learning to overcome my addictions, I learned to change what I like, what I desire, and what I need. You can too. The foundation for making positive changes in your life is retraining the brain. Once you have changed your mind about how you want to live—and when you want to love and nurture yourself—you won't want to put garbage in your body. It's that simple!

Building a High Voltage Life

These days, I've brought my HIGH Voltage workout and eating plan to another level, working one-on-one with many of the world's most fascinating people in the high-profile worlds of beauty, fashion, finance, music, and entertainment. These are people whose fast-paced careers depend not only on looking their best and staying healthy, but also on keeping their energy levels—mental and physical—up!

And once again, what I'm talking about is a lot *deeper* than **JUST A DIET** or **JUST A FITNESS ROUTINE!** It's about reaching down into your soul and getting rid of the negative energy—the **ENERGY BLOCKERS**—that are robbing you of your natural energy, preventing you from achieving whatever it is that you want (and deserve) in life, whether it is . . .

- Losing five pounds—or fifty.
- Finding time to do something for YOURSELF—joining a gym, learning to dance, trying skydiving.
- Freeing yourself from a destructive relationship—with your spouse or lover, your parents, your "best friend," siblings, or even your children.
- Leaving a job . . . starting a new business . . . going back to school . . . or closing a multimillion-dollar megadeal.

Wherever you are in your life, what you feed your brain is equally as important as what you feed your body. They go hand in hand.

I don't *believe in diets. The only kind of diet I believe in is a* **mind diet!**

For years, I channeled my energy into abusing my body and my mind. With drugs. With alcohol. With bingeing and purging in an obsessive desire to stay thin. In the circles that I traveled in when I was married, looking good—meaning thin!—came with the territory (plus I was "paid" *extremely* well for complying!). But I also bought into that "never too rich, never too thin" mentality. I got so good at throwing up, I could do it without smudging my lipstick! When I look back today, it's a miracle I'm still breathing.

They say you have to hit bottom before you start climbing back up—well, I hit bottom so many times that my butt was flat from falling on it. But all that is in the past. And the *only reason* I believe I survived is to be an example for others so that they don't have to go through the same suffering and pain as I did. I'm not merely surviving, either—when people call me a survivor, I take issue with that: this is about surviving and **THRIVING!**

If I Could Get My Totally Dysfunctional Act Together, Anyone Can!

Rediscovering your energy and health, and regaining control over your life (and maybe food-addictive habits), begins with overhauling everything you're putting into your mind and your body.

I can't change your life. But I can show you how YOU can change it—the same way I changed mine.

First off, **START TAKING RESPONSIBILITY.** It makes me crazy when people blame others for their problems. Well, forget about blame. Just forget about it. **IT DOESN'T MATTER.** Whatever you've done, whatever you've experienced, whatever you look like, it doesn't matter as long as you wake up, now!

This is your **wake-up call! YOU** *can get your act together **no matter** what you've done to yourself.*

So, if you've come to the point where you've made the decision that you genuinely want to (or like me, had to!) CHANGE, when you're finally sick and tired of being sick and tired, then now is the hour to reclaim your power!

ENERGY UP! WHOO!

Chapter 2

YOU CAN'T ARGUE WITH SUCCESS!

When I returned to New York, people didn't quite know how to describe me. In fact, I used to get a kick out of it when they said *"What* is that?" rather than *"Who* is that?"

But they tried. Even though I was never part of the "official" health club world (I always created my own little niche), I became known as New York City's hypercharged "Cosmic Queen of Fitness." "Fitness Guru to the Rich and Famous." "Fitness Trainer to the Stars." And "a living Barbie doll." *Vogue* magazine wrote that I was "Fashion's Body Secret" after the total workout/lifestyle overhaul I did for gorgeous model Beverly Peele. She had gained over seventy pounds during her pregnancy, but I had her back on the runway, wowing audiences, a scant eight weeks after her delivery. Of course she had about a hundred thousand ($) good reasons to get back to work real quick—maybe more! And in Australia, *Woman's Day* anointed me "Fitness Priestess to Rock and Movie Stars," after getting an eyeful of music star Dannii Minogue's "total body makeover." Not long after, *I* was thrilled to see that Dannii's controversial *Playboy* spread (October 1995) was a total sellout! Dannii is one of my most dramatic before-and-afters.

I've also been called an "Evangelist for Fitness." I love that one.

Especially when people say that my "energy concerts" are like a cross between a rock concert and
a revival meeting! They are: it's like—hallelujah!

Volt-Note!

In 1986, when writer/social critic Gay Talese wrote
about me for the *New York Times*, he got a kick out
of the fact that my father had been a railroad engi-
neer. Hey, maybe that was the start of my going
WHOOOOOOO! WHOOOOOO! WHOOOOOO!

And you *do* feel uplifted spiritually. Remember
when everyone was talking about "getting into
the zone" when they worked out—experiencing that so-called endorphin
high? Well, there *is* something to it! Those endorphins rushing through your
brain, that energy high you get—they take you to a place that no man-made
drug can. In this life, I believe that God—the universal energy—gives us
everything we need to live in ecstasy—and I don't mean the kind you get in
pill form! I'm talking about the real deal.

　　　Well, that's what I aspire to—that's what I'm about. And that's what
I want for **YOU**. Total energy—total ecstasy. The ability to achieve that is
in each and every one of us. The *New York Times* wasn't kidding when it said
I was like Norman Vincent Peale's brain in Tina Turner's body! So turn on,
tune in, and work out!

The Real Deal

Before I explain how my program will work for you, let me tell you how it's
worked for others. People come to me not only because I'm known for real-
life, real-body results, but because I care. My clients know they can call on
me day and night! The other day I came home to find six messages on my
machine!—including this one from my good friend and client "Downtown"
Julie Brown, MTV's most famous VJ, who's now the host of E! television's
successful celebrity gossip show and, most recently, becoming quite a little
actress.

　　*Voltage! I just wanted to let you know I have been working out like a dog!
　　I've been doing an hour and a half of cardio—the running machine, the
　　bike. I still can't seem to get to your size yet, but my legs are getting thin-*

ner, my body stronger . . . so all I need is the finishing touch—which is you! Hurry up and get out here!

Julie has even adopted and adapted my "Whoo!" to work with her own fantastic style! Traveling with her, you can bet, is always a high-energy trip. People see her—and they go wild. And they should: her warmth and charm—which are real—come right through. I'm so proud of her.

Pop star Taylor Dayne, whose hits include the megaselling "Tell It to My Heart," called me from Los Angeles and told me the news about landing a terrific part in the HBO movie *Stag*—the dramatic female lead—as a stripper! Taylor, cutie pie that she is, has never really had a weight problem, but still didn't feel **TOTALLY** comfortable sauntering around on the big screen in little more than a G-string!—even though that scene was just about thirty seconds long (moviegoers notice everything!). She told me I should get ready to kick her butt **BIG-TIME** to get her in camera-ready shape! Don't forget, on screen, people look eight to ten pounds heavier than they really are! By the way, the movie was a big hit and she got tremendous reviews for her role.

And yes, sometimes a client backslides. Every now and then, super-model Beverly Johnson, one of the great beauties of *all time,* slips and goes on a sugar binge (her weakness: bags of candy!). But I know how to give "good phone." Last time, we talked out her cravings for over an hour! (This is why, if you possibly can, I recommend that you do my program with a friend so you can help each other over the rough spots. A good support system is essential! We'll talk about that a lot more in Chapter Seven).

Even though they know I care, my clients also know that I'm not going to coddle them. With me, you have to be ready for the **REAL DEAL:** daily workouts, sticking to my food plan, no whining, no questions asked! If not, I say go someplace else. I may be caring, but the initials of my company—**DFWM**—that's **DON'T F@#!* WITH ME!**—say it all. Never let it be said, though, that I can't be compassionate. If someone breaks down and starts to cry during a workout, I always wait till they've dried their eyes before I demand thirty more push-ups (just kidding . . . kind of)!

When *Vogue* named me as one of America's 55 Best Personal Trainers, they also said "only for the flamboyant." Maybe so. After all, my first energy concert was in a nightclub for drag queens—who all came dressed as High Voltage! What a compliment! I guess you haven't truly arrived till you're done in drag (*it's a New York thing!*).

People usually come to me through word of mouth, although I've been "won" at a charity auction to which I donated my time, and I've been given as a gift to more high-powered CEOs than I could name, usually for their fortieth or fiftieth birthdays! But until now, for the most part, I've only shared my program with fashion and entertainment industry insiders and others whose livelihoods depend on their staying energetic and in shape. But they believe—and I do too—that it pays to go for the best! Well, I'm proud to say that I'm the highest-paid energy conductor in the country (I'm probably the ONLY one too)!

> **⚡ Volt-Note! ⚡**
>
> **O**ne of the reasons my clients and I forge such close relationships is that so much of my love, and *all* my energy, goes to them. While there is someone who for many years has had a special place in my heart, I always say I have no personal life—my work is my life! The fact is, I'll do **ANYTHING** for my clients but sleep with them (**THAT'S** something **I DON'T** believe in, trendy or not).
>
> For me, sleeping with a client would be like making love with my own child! If my client **NEEDS** a new love, however, I've been known to find them the right person! In fact, my matchmaking has been so on target that quite a few times the match has developed into a long-term relationship. I've even been the guest of honor at a few weddings! I guess I go to any lengths to keep my clients healthy and happy! My motto is—Whatever it takes!

One-on-One and Then Some

Most of the time, I work intensively with a single individual for a few weeks or months to get them ready for an important concert tour, a hot new movie role, or just to energize and revitalize their life. Since I come from a spa background, my specialty is converting my clients' homes, country retreats, and even private islands into spas (our initial, high-intensity "transforming" week—what I call SPA WEEK—is adapted for YOUR High Voltage transformation in Chapter Seven).

I'll admit right here that I'm spoiled. One of my favorite setups is on a yacht. I even have a special "yacht" program that I've devised in which I bring along my own chef and masseuse!—if anyone out there would like to splurge and give it a try, let me know! The only food on board is ours—and it's impossible to sneak off in the middle of the night! One client thought about it, but she realized it would make too much noise to rev up the helicopter!

With private clients, I'm with them 24/7: that means twenty-four hours a day, seven days a week. We work out three to five hours a day, depending on their individual strength and energy level (don't worry, you won't be doing that many hours). If they're not practically comatose by the end of the first day—and walking a bit funny by the second day (from muscles they never knew they had!)—I haven't done my job! Sometimes clients ask me what we do at night during **SPA WEEK.** Well, I just chuckle: the evening activity is crawling into bed and going to sleep!

Keeping Pace—with Yourself!

High Voltage workouts are *high-voltage!* I mean **INTENSE!**—but I haven't lost a client yet. The only person who ever fainted was actor Danny Aiello—but he was fainting on cue in the movie *Key Exchange.* To this day, when he sees me he smiles and yells, "Energy Up! Whoo!"

Besides, whatever I do with clients is geared to their *personal* level of fitness. For some clients, the pace is slower, although it is just as intense to them! One woman, a prominent psychotherapist with loads of natural energy who hadn't exercised in years, was so wiped out after our first warm-up, that a subsequent fifteen minutes on the treadmill had her practically trembling! Afterwards, there was no way I'd let her go into the steam room for fear she *would* pass out.

But she rallied like a trouper, having come to the decision that she wanted her physical energy to match her mental energy. "If I can't get my body moving, how am I ever going to keep up with myself?" she told me. "Sometimes in the evening, I still have a ton of stuff I have to get done, and I'm pooped. I'm convinced that if I'm exercising and eating right, I'll add more hours to my day—for my work, and for my family too!"

My pace is really not that unusual. If you've ever been to a spa, or read about spas in magazines, you know an intense schedule is practically routine. The problem with spas, though, is that no matter how motivated you are when you're there, once you're back in your own environment, you lose that resolve. Your momentum may last a month, but to be honest, you'll be lucky if it lasts as long as a week! It's a problem I struggled to solve for my clients when I was a spa director.

When *I* actually come to my clients' homes, it's a different ball game. I observe firsthand what's causing their stress and their bad eating habits, so I'm able to help them rearrange their lives—and their kitchen cupboards. If there's a chef (and there often is), *my* chef retrains theirs. In fact, I've retrained entire households! More often than you can imagine, people with huge staffs have no one taking proper care of them. I help them stock up on bottled water so there's no excuse for not drinking enough water (an important key to my program). By the way, like many people, I have serious concerns about drinking tap water—and you should too! I hear that lots of new strains of harmful bacteria are showing up in our water these days. A decent filter, which costs anywhere from $10 to $30, can be a smart investment.

My client and I usually start by going away together for several days (I'm a beach baby and I prefer someplace warm, but I'll go anywhere). That's where the real reprogramming takes place. Not long ago, I spent two weeks in Aspen with one of my favorite new clients, let's call him Alan, just thirty years old and already a Grammy Award–winning producer. Blond, a towering six four, and a real sweetheart, Alan had once been a high school jock, but like many young guys, he was so busy building his career that he hadn't done anything physical in years. After working with me, he's fifty pounds lighter, and a **LEAN, MEAN, PUMPING MACHINE!**

Because he practically lives on the road, I personally instructed his chef on how to prepare the meals he takes with him when he flies (is it any surprise to you that I think airline food is a **TOTAL** nightmare!).

But this guy's serious. And he's following *this* leader. In fact, he often checks in with me at the end of the day for suggestions on what to order if he's planning to go out that night! I have to say that he is blessed with tons of his own natural energy; I just helped him reconnect with it. After all, he used to be physically active, but had temporarily lost it. *May I add, he's now yelling, "Energy Up! Whoo!"*

⚡ Volt-Note! ⚡

With Alan, we totally overhauled not only his eating habits, but his entire lifestyle, including his wardrobe (something I do for many of my clients, by the way). Typical of many rock 'n' roll guys, Alan was stuck in a jeans and T-shirt rut. He probably owned more pairs of black jeans than there are days in the month! When I suggested he consider hot designers like Gucci or Dolce & Gabbana, I guess he thought I was talking about a new music act! *But he took my advice and he looks great!*

Not long ago, another favorite client, a gorgeous twenty-six-year-old actress, olive-skinned and exotic, with waist-length shiny black hair (the kind of girl who's so stunning she never pays her own dinner tab!), jetted me down to Miami for a five-day High Voltage recharge. There, at the trendy Delano Hotel in South Beach, we reinforced our "no flour, no sugar, no salt" regime—she had fallen off it for a few months and was up for a big movie part! We also had unbelievable massages and salt-glow treatments at the Agua, the hotel's fabulous women-only penthouse spa. By the end of our stay, my young client looked so terrific she felt *more* than comfortable sashaying around in the steam room and Jacuzzi in front of guests like supermodel Niki Taylor (who, I might add, looked pretty terrific herself after giving birth to twins!).

After spending the initial few days together, I usually head back to a client's own environment and work on incorporating the changes we've made into their everyday lifestyle. If a client has more than one home—and lots do—I like to do my thing at each location. This is the part that clients appreciate the most. As I said, it's not that hard to keep healthy habits while you're away (and especially under my watchful eyes). It's quite another thing to make them standard operating procedure.

It's the Results That Count

The most important thing to me is that my clients get the results they're going for. I recently spent three days getting the "contraband" out of the kitchen of a drop-dead handsome young banker, just in his early thirties, who was in the middle of building an awesome "medieval" castle in

Southampton, Long Island. I also developed a rigorous workout for him to match the one I created for his girlfriend, who is one of my longtime clients.

Model Beverly Johnson (who, like me, went through her own bouts with bulimia—and has courageously written and spoken about it too) lost a quick twenty pounds following my program. I've also worked out with her pretty teenage daughter Anansa, helping to prepare her for a modeling career. As for Dieter Esch, owner of the Wilhelmina agency (one of New York's most prestigious modeling agencies), he dropped forty-one pounds once I got him to cut flour, sugar, and salt out of his diet.

A typically macho guy, Dieter was a tough case when it came to accepting my "follow the leader" bit—especially since it was coming from a wild woman who he probably thought looked like she was from Mars! Sitting behind his big, imposing desk, he was a bit stunned by my appearance and attitude, to say the least. But that's often the response I get from very powerful men. First, they're perplexed; then they usually break out in a grin. But they also realize *very quickly* that there's nothing sexual going on. In fact, when we work together, clients are more likely to end up saluting me than coming on to me.

Following the Leader

All of my clients learn that when I say "follow the leader," I mean it—especially for my three

---

~~ **Volt-Note!** ~~

By the way, when his castle is finished, everyone will be able to admire my handiwork, considering that in the middle of the swimming pool is a nude statue of his girlfriend—my client—costumed as a mermaid! Anatomically correct too (up to the fin, that is!). I may be prejudiced, but they really are one of the best-looking couples I have ever seen! Also the sweetest!

~~ **Volt-Note!** ~~

Of course, I always ask my clients about any physical limitations they may have, such as knee or back injuries, as well as about any allergies and any medications or hormones they may be taking that might affect their progress (when a client is on hormones for any reason, be it the birth control pill, estrogen replacement therapy, or whatever, I know we're in for a slower ride down the scales). Michelle, fifty-five, a supersuccessful real estate broker (known for her sales of homes of the rich and famous), was one client whose body seemed stuck, even on my program: it just wouldn't let go of the extra weight (and she was anxious to be in supershape for her daughter's wedding just a few months down the line). That's when I turned into supersleuth. "Don't worry," I told her. "Whatever it is, it can be dealt with. We're going to play detective and I promise you, I will not stop till I find out what the hell is going on!" (I'm like a little pit bull—when I get hold of something, I won't let go!) Scratch tests from her nutritionist finally revealed a food allergy—to potatoes!—which we quickly took into consideration. (By the way, she turned out to be one truly beaming mother of the bride!)

nonnegotiable rules—no flour, no sugar, no salt. I find that even though my clients are all successful, high-powered people, they're totally cool about giving over their power to me. After all, they make decisions all day in reference to the part of their life that works—usually their careers. They're coming to me for something they know doesn't work, and they're more than ready and willing to try it MY WAY.

Jumping the Hurdles

One of the coolest clients I ever had was Linda, an ultrabusy executive who ran a **MAJOR** foundation, had a huge, art-filled Fifth Avenue apartment straight out of *Architectural Digest,* was happily married with two gorgeous kids—she had it all! (Although she had a full staff, she even managed to do a lot of her own cooking and housekeeping—a real mensch!)

When we first met, Linda balked a bit at cutting *all* flour from her diet. Bread was her weakness. But once she did, she was so thrilled with a practically immediate six-pound weight loss (all she really needed to lose) that the flour has stayed out to this day—no backsliding.

Linda simply incorporated my "no flour, no kidding" rule into her daily life. All I had to say to her was, "Take a piece of bread, chew it up, spit it out in your hand, place it on your thighs—'cause that's exactly where it's going! It doesn't even stop in your stomach," and that did it for her. She's never been able to look at a piece of bread the same way since!

Novelist Tama Janowitz likes to joke that she was "very close to death" after she first attempted my workout in 1994, shortly before her book *The Male Cross-Dresser Support Group* was published (a follow-up to her big best-seller, *Slaves of New York*). Of course, her idea of exercise before meeting me was sitting in bed eating bonbons! Her mother assured me that I was the only person on the planet who could get her daughter to move, as I prepared Tama for her book tour. With Tama, we were clearly dealing with more of an energy issue than a weight issue. (Like Linda, Tama only wanted to lose five or six pounds—she's actually naturally thin!) But I tend to specialize in people who hate to work out. The difference is, I make it fun!

Since then, Tama and I have been great buddies! The following year,

I helped get her in shape for a two-week horseback trip through the Indian region of Rajasthan for an assignment she was doing for *Travel & Leisure* magazine. She says she brought me on board to get her thighs in shape for all that riding; I always say she paid me to make her miserable for two and a half hours a day, because she knew it was the only way she was going make it through that trip! (These days, when we talk, I kid her that I don't want to be interrupting her workout time! But her energy must be up, because she's looking great—plus she just adopted a beautiful baby girl. Now she's doing exercises using her daughter as a weight!)

I've already mentioned pop star and up-and-coming actress Taylor Dayne, a longtime client and dear friend. Now, Taylor has a great body, but always thinks that she's a little bit bottom-heavy (of course, even I think I'm a little bottom-heavy—so go figure!). When she first heard "no flour, no sugar, no salt," she thought I was f@#!*ing nuts—and said so (many people do!). But Taylor's a no-nonsense girl—and on her frame, eight to ten pounds make a difference. In 1995, when we went out to her beautiful Long Island estate for a five-day **SPA WEEK,** those pounds (and inches, I may add) came right off, and she changed her tune. And we all know Taylor can carry a high note! She's got a voice that's a powerhouse!

One of the hardest things for Taylor to accept was that the *tiny* bit of alcohol she indulged in (I'm talking a glass of wine every now and then) could be a problem. But many people swell up from even the smallest amounts of alcohol (not to mention that drinking makes it easier to make bad food choices that you wouldn't otherwise).

Eventually Taylor came around. They *all* do. When she deviates from our program, of course, the weight sneaks back on. But then I'll hear from her and we'll take a little spa weekend for a High Voltage tune-up.

It's not often that I get a client who questions my bottom line—no pun intended. I don't really work with people who are resistant—otherwise they wouldn't be hiring me for the kind of big bucks they shell out. By the time people come to me, they know the score, know what I'm about, are serious about the time and effort they're going to give me, and are willing to pay the price.

Occasionally, though, I get a hard case. There was the high-powered

West Coast CEO who purchased a week with me from a charity auction for his wife. To my delight, I was whisked off to California and ensconced in a magnificent guest house (which I'd be more than happy to make my permanent residence!) on their Bel Air estate. This was the usual client lap of luxury—huge staff, sumptuously decorated interiors, a home gym so well equipped that it practically rivaled the best health club you could imagine (and remember, I don't like gyms; the lighting usually sucks and they smell funny!).

The client, Katherine, was pretty, with perfectly cut, shoulder-length blond hair, and conservative by nature. I guess I looked like a blown-up Barbie doll to her! She was slightly overweight (by High Voltage standards, that is), and really didn't have any major energy blocks—her fairy tale life suited her just fine, thank you. Still, she was just a little curious about what I could teach her about staying in shape. Once we found a common denominator (our mutual love of dancing), I flatter myself that I won her over and even opened her eyes to some new ways of thinking.

energy up!

Volt-Note!

Despite this family's wealth and privilege, their eating habits were a bit dysfunctional, due in part to an old-school French chef who was practically wedded to butter, eggs, and cream! Although Katherine never thought he would tolerate criticism, I just kept explaining to him, over and over, that when it came to the family's health, energy, and well-being, he was the most important person in the household. (Plus, underneath it all, I suspect he wanted to shed a few pounds too!)

Water, My Drink of Choice

Another issue that often encounters a *little* resistance is the amount of water I ask my clients to drink: at least six to eight eight-ounce bottles of water a day. For some reason, drinking from little bottles is much easier than drinking from glasses!

Now, eight glasses of water a day is not an outlandish amount—once you get used to it! In fact, most spas, health clubs, nutritionists (and even doctors, surprise, surprise!) recommend pretty much the same thing. But I am *serious* about it—the more you drink, the more you lose! (By the way, I don't drink water with my meals, which goes back to an old spa theory that it interferes with digestion. Whether that's true or not, I really don't know. But it works for me.)

When someone hires me, we always have plenty of water at hand: as soon as you're finished gulping down one bottle, there I am with another! I'm constantly handing out water bottles! The only downside to all this water is that you *do* have to spend a lot of time in the bathroom! For those of us who came through the drug era, time spent in the bathroom (we were either snorting up or throwing up, back then) is no big deal.

I work hard with my clients to help take their minds off any negative energy they may be dealing with. The more negative or resistant they are, the harder I work to pull them through. But the moment they start feeling better, they become less resistant. I always say, when you start yelling "Energy Up! Whoo!" with me, I've got you—or better, **YOU'VE** got you!

Even the **Stars** Have **Trouble** with **French Fries!**

I first met Downtown Julie Brown on the set of *Club MTV*, where I was part of a special fashion segment. (To tell you the truth, it was more *"flashion"* than fashion—that's the High Voltage word for clothes decked out in glitter, pearls, and rhinestones! And I love it! I used to say that rhinestones are the only way that High Voltage gets "stoned" anymore.)

> **Volt-Note!**
>
> What I'm actually doing is reprogramming—creating a blueprint for new, healthy patterns in life. Sometimes when people start with me, they get caught up in the Voltage image. But after we spend a little time together, it suddenly dawns on them that this is a serious endeavor we're taking on—a real commitment—and that I'm just trying to make it as entertaining and pleasant as possible!

Julie was very quick to tell me—in her adorable English accent—that she was practically living on baskets of french fries. Julie, who everybody knows has a sleek and sexy little shape, admits to a tendency to plump up a bit when she isn't being absolutely careful. But after she went on my intensive program—a five-week energy marathon!—she was in the best shape of her life! She never felt better, **LOOKED MORE GORGEOUS,** or had more energy (and anyone who knows Julie knows that could be good or bad!). I think that if we discovered that certain foods gave *me* more energy, people would say, "Don't eat them, Voltage!"

Dannii Minogue, widely regarded as a national treasure in England and her native Australia (and who just signed a big recording contract with Warner

Records!), is another of my best success stories. Dannii practically grew up in the public eye. As an adolescent she became as familiar to Australians as the Mouseketeers are to audiences here. Next, she went on to star in a popular soap opera (as did her big sister, pop star Kylie); then she followed her sister into the highly visible music biz.

Dannii was only seventeen when we first met. With her creamy skin and mesmerizing blue eyes, she looked like a little angel (she's just five feet two inches tall!). But she was plagued by what I could see was only "baby fat," and needed someone to get her on the right track.

Since then, Dannii's totally transformed herself. In fact, she's probably my most disciplined, most centered client. After a big TV show or road tour, she may have put on a pound or two, but she's always quick to snap back (this is certainly her lifestyle of choice!). Whenever Dannii is in New York, we meet for a spa-style pick-me-up. When she married the ex–Prime Minister's son, I was flown out to Melbourne to help get her ready for her wedding!

I can imagine what you're thinking. Yachts. Fancy hotel spas. Private islands. Private chefs. Is this sort of routine realistic for most people? No way! But while some people may find all this luxury intimidating, I think it's better to take inspiration from it! And come on, I couldn't afford me either! (No wonder I like to work all the time, it's the only way I can afford my lifestyle!) But don't forget, my clients often have million-dollar recording contracts and movie deals riding on how they look.

I have to say, I really love working with clients who have strong motivation like this (*we should all have that sort of motivation!*). They take everything I say and use it to the hilt.

Of course, it's easier to take what I say with open arms when you've got to be back on the runway or ready for a film in a few short weeks or months. But these same formulas work for everyone! Trust me! Besides, everybody needs energy—to cope with jobs, school, families, to be able to handle whatever is going on round the clock in your life! Remember, all the world's a stage—and on *your* stage, *you* play the starring role!

The Real Food Scoop

I want to change your mind about food, and you'll discover that it's not as hard as it seems. For example, some of the High Voltage principles I'm going to tell you about in the pages ahead may be easy for you to understand, but I know that some of you may be so brainwashed with the current stupid diet thinking that you may find some of my ideas hard to accept.

However, check this out:

- Who's going to argue that it's *not* a good thing to drink six to eight glasses of water a day and to eat as close to nature as possible?
- Who's going to say that sugar is good for you?
- Who's going to champion limp, overprocessed canned or frozen veggies over crisp, fresh-from-the-garden produce?
- Is there anyone out there who wants to argue that chemicals, unpronounceable additives, preservatives, and the other junk that you find in processed food are *good* things? (My rule: If you can't spell it—or can't pronounce it—don't put it in your mouth!)

I know that "no flour" is the toughest hurdle for most people. But there's no question that flour is the worst energy zapper there is: it puffs you up like a balloon till you're walking around like the Pillsbury Doughboy (I always say, keep eating those Pillsbury products and you'll look just like him too). Eliminating flour from your diet produces dramatic—often immediate—results in terms of weight loss. No, I don't know how it works—only that it does! I think of flour as a "thickener." If you do any cooking, you know what I'm saying—flour is what you use to thicken gravies and sauces, right? So who wants to use it to thicken their body?

I'm going to change some of your other ideas too. For instance, some foods that you've been told are acceptable, like pasta, are actually **DEADLY** to Voltage eating—especially *if* you happen to be a food addict like me!

Pasta is made from flour, one of the most addictive foods around.

Still, we all know someone who is skinny as a rail and who practically lives on pasta, right? (Well, more power to them, but if that's not you, so what?) Every *body* is different! I read recently that twenty-five percent of the population can eat anything they want and not gain weight (wow!), twenty-five percent have a hard time with carbohydrates and sugars (like me!), and the rest of you are somewhere in between (i.e., some carbs you can eat, like popcorn and rice; some you can't). It's a little like being lactose-intolerant (unable to digest milk). You can be violently allergic . . . or just get a bit gassy. Think about where you might fall in.

- Do you start each day with coffee and a bagel (or a muffin, toast, or a Danish)?
- Would you rather eat bread than dessert? Is the thought of life without bread devastating?
- Have you ever finished off a whole package of crackers or cookies by yourself, without even realizing it?
- Would you find it difficult to prepare dinner for a week without relying on pizza or pasta?

If you've answered yes to any of these questions, I can bet that flour may be your trigger.

The Fat-Free Food Scam

I want to add a word here about all those fat-free foods and treats that are filling the supermarket shelves. And that word is: **GARBAGE!** What a scam! Fat-free products often have the same number of calories that regular products do! And while they may have no fat, they usually have plenty of sugar and salt (the taste has to come from somewhere!).

So why is it that women especially seem to think that since Snack-Well's cookies are fat-free, they can eat the whole box? Not only will you not lose any weight on those things, but you'll probably end up *gaining* weight. Fat-free treats often do people more harm than good!

If I haven't seen one of my clients for a while, and he or she comes back to me ten or even fifteen pounds heavier, I always say: "Don't tell me—

you went on the fat-free diet!" And they can't believe that I can tell *exactly* what it is that they've been cheating on.

Well, I'm not psychic, sweetie pie, but come on! Open up those cabinets and kitchen cupboards and there it is! Entenmann's fat-free marshmallow iced devil's food cake. Or fat-free fudge brownies. Mind you, these are intelligent, successful people who have just temporarily bought into advertising hype! Thank God, in a matter of days, we're usually back on track.

What Voltage Can Do for You!

If you've lost that last ten pounds at least ten times, gone from Scarsdale to Slim-Fast, and are ready to put yourself in my hands, follow my lead, allow me to change your relationship to food (how you eat, why you eat, what you eat), and follow my three nonnegotiable principles (no white flour, no sugar, no salt, no kidding!) *and get your body moving*—I mean exercising, the High Voltage way, every day, for at least a week—at the end of that week, I promise that you'll be feeling better, feeling lighter, and more energized than you've ever felt in your life. *And, once you feel that way and know what I'm all about, you'll be ready to* stay with the program *for the weeks ahead.*

You see, my darlings, as I said before, my job is to get you to where you can eat anything you want—it's just that what you want will change dramatically. Trust me: this is not about strengthening your willpower or learning to live with being hungry or deprived.

At the same time—**AND THIS IS IMPORTANT!**—it's also **NOT** about trying to make your present formula work or fitting this program into your life and its existing patterns.

If that's what you're trying to do, you might as well stop right here. **THIS IS ABOUT FUNDAMENTALLY CHANGING YOUR LIFE** (for the better) and **CHANGING THOSE PATTERNS** (to healthy, life-enhancing ones). You know what they say, if it ain't broke, don't fix it? Well—**NEWS FLASH, AMERICA!—IT'S BROKE!**

I wish I could come into each and every one of your homes and work with you personally. It's fun having me around—or so my clients tell me! But this book is my vehicle for doing just that. If you're a food addict (like me, like so many of my clients), imagine the relief you're going to feel when you get through your first few days not thinking about food in the same old way. Imagine how good it's going to feel not wanting to gorge on cupcakes, pies, or bread—or hating yourself because you did. Think about how it's going to be not to live in guilt . . . or feel deprived (God, I hate that word!). That is **NOT** what High Voltage is about!

So forget about diet books and fitness books—you know they're bullshit. Forget about counting fat grams and tricky food combinations. That just doesn't work. But be forewarned: If you're a veteran of the diet wars, and have tried everything else, **ENERGY UP!** is different from anything else you've ever tried (and tried and tried!). And it's not easy (nothing ever is)—although I try to make it as easy and joyful as possible. But there is no magic bullet. The only magic bullet is the promise I can give you (borrowing the words of the legendary women's rights champion Susan B. Anthony): **"FAILURE IS IMPOSSIBLE."** If you really give in to it and enjoy it, it will work.

But with my promise of results, you have to give me yours for commitment. If you don't want to become a statistic—getting fatter and more unhappy, aging miserably (not joyfully!)—you have to be ready to change not just the way you eat, but the way you **THINK!** And you can do it, if you'll just **GET WITH THE PROGRAM!**

There is a lot of great stuff that comes with being fifty years old. And I am glad that I can share my five decades of experience with you, because I am still going strong and I want you to feel the way I feel (hey, in addition to changing bodies here, maybe we can change some tired ideas about aging in the bargain!).

So, if you're ready to embrace it—**TAKE A STAND, JOIN THE COSMIC COMMAND, AND YELL:**

ENERGY UP! WHOO!

Chapter 3

RECHARGING YOUR MENTAL BATTERIES

n my heart and soul I have always felt that there is an energy crisis on this planet—and that I'm here to help turn the power back on. When I see someone shuffling (not striding) down the street, with her head down, shoulders slumped, eyes devoid of inner light, I want to run after her, hug her, and shout, **"ENERGY UP! WHOO!"** After all, energy is what we *all* want; it's what this book is *really* about: how to get it, how to keep it, how to make it work for you. "Energy is like a muscle," I tell my clients. "If you don't use it, you lose it." And I don't want **YOU** to lose it either. So let me tell you first about the techniques I use to discover what's blocking my clients' energies—and then how you can apply them to get your own energy recharged.

Energy is what gets us moving. It's what makes us able to wake up in the morning, happy to be alive. Are you excited? Well, energy is having excitement about life! It's sidewalk-fair exuberance—it's the tool you need to experience life on this planet to the fullest without being hung up on negative feelings, fear, or sorrow. Energy is when you wake up and go Whoo!—feel great about yourself and just can't wait to get going!

I wake up each and every morning and run and kiss myself in the mirror, over and over again. I say, "Voltage—I really love you, you're the sweetest!" And I mean it! I crack me up. I entertain me. Silly? Maybe . . .

but I do it anyway. **IT KEEPS ME CONNECTED TO MY SELF-LOVE, WHICH IS THE CORE PHILOSOPHY OF THIS BOOK!**

Right now, though, you probably can't feel it, can't get it, and can't live, move, and breathe in a high-energy way. You can't enter the **VOLT**-Age when you're still plagued by energy blockers—*negative* emotions (like jealousy, fear, resentment, or frustration) that are stopping you from putting your *positive* energy forward in your work, in your relationships, and in your life. So, besides changing your mind about food and about exercise, I am going to change your mind. Period. It's been said before, but in order to change your life, you've got to change your mind first.

⚡ Volt-Note! ⚡

Be careful of anyone who promises that they're going to give you energy . . . because it's just not theirs to give (just as it's not mine to give either). Energy is universal—it exists free for every human being on earth. As far as I am concerned, anyone can tune in or turn on to the energy force that runs this planet.

Turn On the Energy Channel

How do I turn on a new client's energy? How can you turn on yours? Let me take you through the steps.

When I work with a new client, the most important thing I do is OBSERVE. First, I look at the obvious. How are they dressed? Prim and proper? Overtly sexy or plain Jane? People send out messages about themselves with their clothing and their attitudes.

Put On a Happy Face . . .

I notice facial expressions: a lot of people have turned-down, gloomy looks. So when they come to me like that, one of the first things I ask them to do is smile! (I smile a lot—my energy comes from internal happiness. Plus, it's a family trait. My sister should be doing toothpaste commercials!)

But believe it or not, some people actually feel uncomfortable smiling. When I put a mirror in front of them and say, "Now smile. Look joyful!"—they don't even know what I'm talking about. Some people are just uncomfortable with being happy and they don't even realize it. I say, "Can't you just smile because you're happy to be alive? You woke up today. You have a roof over your head. You have someone around that cares about you."

People like that sometimes need a reality check—and a shot of High Voltage—big-time!

Try it yourself right now. Get up and go to a mirror and *smile*. I'll be surprised if it doesn't change the way you feel.

. . . But Watch the Makeup!

Makeup tells a lot about a woman too. Some women haven't changed their style in a decade or more. You've seen them: women who are still wearing their makeup (or doing their hair!) the way they did when they felt they were at their sexiest and most youthful. *But* sometimes, your exterior look reflects your interior energy; when it gets stuck—not moving or changing—you get stuck too!

Outdated makeup is one of the small energy blockers I notice, but wearing too much makeup is another. I know about that firsthand, because I've lived it firsthand. Before I had my face done—recharged my packaging—I was piling on makeup **BIG-TIME.** But too much makeup and you start looking like an aging drag queen! Think back to when you were a teenager and why you first started to wear makeup in the first place: to look *older,* right? Well, it still works that way! So lighten up!

When in Doubt, Throw It Out!

Updating your style is definitely an energy booster, and it's something I get involved in with clients. I go shopping with them; I go through their closets and get rid of stuff they haven't worn in years. I want you to do this too (get a friend to help you out).

My thing is to get rid of clutter—in your closets, sure, but also in your thoughts and your

Volt-Note

Sometimes I have clients keep a "relic" from their closet (a pair of size 6 suede pants you haven't been able to squeeze into in years can be real motivating factor!). But once you get your weight down—and maintain it for three months—get rid of those too big clothes. 'Cause if you keep 'em, you're going to grow back into 'em. I've had clients who have four wardrobes—**COMPLETE**—in four sizes. **BIG MISTAKE!** Keep your wardrobe simple. I always say I don't need a million-dollar wardrobe—I've got a million-dollar body! *And any body can too!*

33

life—and this is one way to start. Clutter drains your energy. Papers piling up. Old magazines you're never going to read. Clothes stuffed into drawers. Things in piles everywhere. I say: **DEPRESSING!** Do you have too much clutter around you, holding you back? I once did. But I'll never be trapped by my trappings again. Today, I have trimmings. **IT'S A MUCH BETTER DEAL**. **GET REAL!**

Atten-shun!

I also notice how clients carry themselves: posture is a factor that clues me in on energy level and self-esteem. Of course, bad posture is practically applauded in the modeling world. But models who slouch stylishly down the runway soon learn that the same thing doesn't look at all attractive in real life. Years ago, when I would slip backstage during fashion shows, I'd see some of the fashion industry's most famous faces, slumped in their chairs, cigarettes in one hand, bagels in the other. Since I'm known for my super-erect posture—I was raised to be a figure skater (and became a figure-skating champion!) and was taught to stand up straight from a very early age—the minute the girls would see me, they'd eye each other, and immediately straighten up!

Off the fashion runways, rounded slumpy shoulders (which can contribute to pouchy abs and a host of back problems) can be a sign of lack of confidence. When someone starts to work with me, we work on that: I'm constantly saying, "Stomach tight, buttocks tight, tuck it in, tuck it under!" Make this one of your mantras too—every time you catch yourself slumping (when you walk down the street, try to catch a glimpse of yourself in the store windows). It's hard to be depressed when you're standing up tall, shoulders up, back, and down. Carry yourself proudly, then try being depressed. It doesn't work!

Do You Hear What I Hear?

And then, I listen. The tone of someone's voice, the authority (or lack of authority!) with which they speak, tells me what they truly think about themselves, It's not *what* you say sometimes, it's *how* you say it. Do you sound tired and depressed? Does your voice lack energy, vitality, and vigor? Are people always asking you to "speak up"? I want you to sound as good as you're going to look.

The next thing I do is talk with the client: as we spend the day together. In the course of walking on the beach, working out, or taking a break for a steam or sauna (a lot of truth comes out when you're buck naked!). Of course, when I talk with a client, it's **TOTALLY** different from their talking to a therapist or their best friend. Maybe their career isn't going the way they think it should. Maybe their manager or agent isn't doing a good job for them. We may get into serious stuff (I'm trying to get them to **THINK** about their lives!), but I make them laugh. I'm tough—but I do my hardest work with a smile. Note: To do this kind of assessment at home, check out the energy blocker quizzes in this chapter, beginning on page 46.

Being Open to Change

Of course, I have to work with different clients in different ways. Sometimes I have to feel around to get a read on their personality. Are they stubborn? Are they resistant in certain areas? One wildly successful TV star whose slinky brunette good looks have graced the covers of almost every magazine you can think of had a manager/boyfriend who was handsome and energetic, but *totally incompatible* with her. Although I could see it was troubling her, I could also see it was something that she wasn't ready to admit to herself, let alone to me. Her relationship was a subject I stayed away from until she was ready to bring it up. You have to find out which buttons to push—and when—to make someone **OPEN** to change.

Obviously this can sometimes be a challenge—but I love a challenge! (This is where I apply my Ph.D. in common sense, University of the Streets.) It's almost like plotting a chess game, checking out the situation, knowing when to advance, when to pull back—but **NOT** a game played with the idea of winning or losing or checkmate. This is not about ego for me, sweetie. I am not here to exert my power and make a point that I can get **ANYBODY**

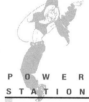

P O W E R
S T A T I O N

HIGH

VOLTAGE

IS A LOT

OF FUN.

HIGH

VOLTAGE

IS FOR

EVERY-

ONE.

TO DO ANYTHING. Then the process wouldn't be fun—it would be a battle all the time. And High Voltage is fun!

I don't force clients into anything, however. I've discovered that my clients **WANT** to tap into something they feel I have—or that I've been able to tap into (I always say it's not me—it's just that universal energy that I'm part of!).

Not Everyone's Ready to Change!

Before I take on someone new, I interview them first. They think they're interviewing me (hah!), but when we're done I let them know the truth, which most people find pretty funny!

The questions I ask depend on the individual. I want to know if they're really ready to change (so we don't waste my time—or theirs). I want to know *what* they want to change in their lives—and even more important, *why*. Is it for them? Is it for someone else? Will it make them happier? Healthier? Wealthier? *Whatever!*

I also need to know if the client's expectations of what I can help them do are based in reality (even if it's only mine!). Are their goals doable in the amount of time we have together? And am I the right person for them? Sometimes not . . . and I've sent them to other people or places. I'm proud to say that usually the first impression I arrive at—part intuition, part conversation, and part revelation—is right on target.

I am willing to work with just about everyone, but on occasion, if I sense that the person is not ready to make a fundamental change, or that I'm not going to enjoy the process with them, I'll pass (after all, what I do is very personal and there are only so many hours in the day). Plus, if I sense certain kinds of resistance, I just may be "too busy" to take them on.

You Wear What You Eat!

Without asking, I can usually tell what my clients are eating just by the way they look. Bulges. Bloating. Fingers and hands that are swollen and puffy. *It's pretty obvious that it's flour, sugar, or salt—one, or all, of the above!*

If they've got a lot of cellulite, for example—that's usually a result of eating flour and salt. (Of course, as I always say, some cellulite is just hereditary—I swear to God, even I have some, although most people think I'm the only one who can see it. Trust me, I don't eat **ANY** flour.)

Clients don't undress when we meet (a woman may pull up her skirt and show me her butt; a guy may pick up his shirt and let me poke his abs), but that's about it. I'm very touchy-feely too, but believe me, it's just not done in a sexual way. It's more like a poke here, a poke there. Just like people poking my abs when I go out—or poking my breasts ever since they've been redone (there's just something about them that's so outrageous they're **FUN!** Everyone wants to touch them! Like I said, I should have done it years ago!).

You are what you eat. Everything you put in your mouth shows up on your body, somewhere.

So take a good, long, honest look in a full-length mirror. Excess cellulite? That usually tells me that pasta, breads, and salty foods, and perhaps even carbonated sodas, are a big part of your diet. Swollen fingers and a general, unhealthy puffiness, especially around the face and eyes? It could be alcohol (for some people, even as little as a glass of wine a day can cause puffiness). Or too much salt that you may not even be aware of (not necessarily from snack foods or french fries, but hidden in salad dressings, cheese, soups, and prepared or packaged foods).

Once you start becoming aware of the fact that your body is built on what you put into it, you'll think twice about your next bacon cheeseburger, pepperoni pizza, or fried food.

It Has to Click!

I have never worked with anyone who was actually *ecstatic* when I told them everything we were going to do, from my well-

> ### Volt-Note!
> Sometimes clients are surprised that other than asking if they smoke cigarettes, I don't really address the smoking issue with them. As an ex-smoker who stopped smoking over twenty years ago, I find that once you're on my program, and you're into treating your body well, smoking falls by the wayside, naturally. Very seldom do any of my clients who follow the High Voltage way keep smoking in their lives. This goes for the current cigar fad too, by the way. I find it so comical that a lot of otherwise fabulous women are puffing away at those phallic things. That's just not the way I would assert my fabulousness, elegance, or power, or whatever it is they think they're doing. It's like playing follow-the-leader in a negative way.

known no flour, no sugar, no salt, no alcohol rulings to the unrelenting pace of our workouts! To be honest, normally they're either shaking, crying, or very upset!

One dinner I will never forget took place on an idyllic Caribbean island with a lovely up-and-coming actress who was very attached to food. Sitting down to our first dinner together, I looked up and saw a tear trickling down her pretty face as she gazed at her plate of grilled fish and salad—but no bread, no wine, none of the extras she was accustomed to. "Baby, what's the matter?" I asked—and the floodgates opened! "I don't know if I can do this," my client wailed. Startled, I reassured her that her way didn't work—or she wouldn't be sitting across from me!

Still, once clients start **GETTING** what I'm talking about—once it clicks—they start fundamentally changing how they think about things. I may be starting to sound like a broken record, but that's how we change the tapes in your head. Reinforcement. Repetition. That's how we get you to where you're going to want to do only the things that are good for you—which you will, after reading this book!

That's What Being an Energy Conductor Is All About!

I'm also changing perceptions, pointing out different ways of looking at things, opening up my clients' eyes to the possibilities of new ways of thinking (yes, I admit it, there's a strong metaphysical streak here!). Because of what I've been through in *my* life, I believe that everything that you experience you're *meant* to experience. There is no such thing as "bad"—you learn from everything that happens . . . and if you don't learn, you're going to keep having the same problems, over and over. Unfortunately most people don't learn from their mistakes; they keep on fine-tuning the same mistakes, again and again and again.

As Gloria Steinem Said, "This Is What Fifty Looks Like."

Fear of aging can be a big energy blocker. Many people are so frightened about getting older that the emotion overwhelms everything else that is positive in their lives. I've had clients tell me, "I don't feel good anymore," "I don't feel the way—or look the way—I did when I was younger," and even, "I'm not as sexy—but that's okay because I'm older." This makes me nuts because once you find a reason to justify feeling "less" than you used to, then you become resigned and accept the condition as fact.

Well, I say, f@#!* that. Forget about aging negatively. You don't have to get out of shape. You don't have to lose your sex appeal. You don't have to lose your zest and energy for life! If anything, you can be stronger and more vibrant (and boy, do I get funny looks from people when I make comments like that!). But when someone asks, "What makes your program so different?"—I say, "Well, you're looking at it! This is what fifty years old looks like. And I'll be saying the same thing when I'm sixty!"

I was so impressed about a decade ago when Gloria Steinem, the famous—and glamorous—feminist writer, turned fifty and coined the phrase "This is what fifty looks like." It's something I say a lot today. She and I happened to meet many years ago when we were both guests at New Age Health Farm, a health retreat in upstate New York where she went every year with her sister. During the few weeks we were there, I always felt that we really bonded. (I'm still a huge fan, even though we haven't spoken in years!)

I am a living example of my principles. I am fifty years old—and I've been doing this for a long time: I know what I'm talking about! I've been as up as anybody can be, and I've been as down as anybody can be, but I've never let my setbacks turn into negativity (I take them as learning experiences).

Of course, I've had lapses too. About ten years ago, I let a bad relationship drag me down—not to the depths that I was in the first time around, but I wasn't my High Voltage self either. I even "forgot" I was an addictive personality and stopped following my own formulas! But boy, I follow them to the letter today!—I have to and I want to. I'm an obsessive, addictive, compulsive personality and this book is dedicated to the millions upon millions of others like me on this planet.

The Naked Truth

I'm nonchalant about nudity because I'm not approaching it from a sexual point of view (don't let my boobs fool you there!). Besides, what could be more natural than to get naked in a steam room or sauna—or to take a good hard look at your own body when you're working with a trainer to whom you're paying top dollar?

Sometimes, though, my forthrightness surprises clients. They don't always realize that whatever they do, I do—from working out with them to . . . whatever! Since my usual routine is to stick with a client 24/7 (I literally wake them up in the morning and tuck them in at night!), I had no qualms at all about shimmying out of my workout gear and following one client—forty-three, good-looking, and literally one of the most powerful men in Boston—right into his steam room. Although he is rather worldly, he admits he was a bit shaken (I don't think he had ever been in a room with a naked woman with whom he wasn't going to have sex!). To this day, it's a story he tells over and over at fancy Back Bay dinner parties!

Still, when people are nervous with nudity, I often take it as a red flag that a body-image energy block exists. I remember one of my clients, a gorgeous young woman from a prominent Chicago family, whose body was FF by the time I was done with her (**FF** stands for *F@#!*ING FIERCE* in Voltage language). She surprised me by wearing her bra and panties into the steam room. That's like wearing a parka at a nude beach! I later learned that she felt self-conscious about her breasts—which she thought were too big—and no one but her boyfriend had ever seen her undressed! After a few days together, working out and discussing her hang-ups and insecurities, she actually felt comfortable enough to relax with me *au naturel* in an outdoor Jacuzzi (at the tip of a cliff overlooking Los Angeles!), much to her boyfriend's amazement—and delight!

Overcoming Your Energy Blockers

Issues that block your energy can be on-the-job problems—like a boss who makes you so depressed that you reach for a candy bar every afternoon. Or a schedule that leaves you so emotionally and physically zapped that all you can do when you get home is phone out for a greasy pizza—with extra cheese. An unfulfilling work life—in which you're underappreciated and underpaid—can be a *nightmare*, draining energy out of every aspect of your life, from your mental outlook to the way you walk and move. When you're down, people know it: they can see tension and depression in the lines of your face.

And let me tell you—if, like most people's, your life includes the demands of a spouse and kids on top of your job, and it's you that keeps it all going, sweetie pie, *you've got to keep your energy up!*

If you don't take care of yourself, sooner or later you're going to be drained of ALL your energy, physical and spiritual. It always amazes me when people comment about *my* energy. Well, I don't know how *YOU* do it! I look forward to going home every night, unplugging my phone, and talking to no one! I have enormous respect for all those women who do it all. In fact, I salute you!—and I'm here to help you hold it all together!

What's Shorting Your Circuits?

An energy block can center on relationships—the demands of parents or a child, a so-called "best friend" who's always putting you down, or daily battles with your teenage daughter who thinks sticking to a curfew means coming home at two A.M.!

Or it could be a boyfriend, a lover or significant other with whom you're just not connecting anymore. Do his eyes seem to wander toward every little sweetie with a navel ring? Or is he suddenly seeing his ex "just as a friend" these days? How about a spouse who's always preoccupied with work? But think about this issue carefully. When you say he takes you for granted, do you mean not thanking you for ironing his shirts, or does he ignore your hopes, your dreams, your very existence?

There's no question that a bad relationship with a boyfriend, lover, or spouse can sit on your spirit and drain you totally! One of my clients, a smart, sexy, and successful forty-year-old, a real player in the advertising biz, who just came out of a verbally abusive relationship (and grueling divorce), agrees: "I was never so totally low-energy as when I was with Michael," she remembers. "I wasn't overweight, but I looked lousy. A few weeks after I left him, I started looking pretty again. I even stood straighter."

Everyone is aware that positive energy is infectious—but so is negative energy! I have noticed that my clients' boyfriends and husbands often get nervous when I'm around, and rightly so. I can't tell you how many times I've helped my clients **HELP THEMSELVES** by getting rid of lovers, husbands, bosses, who were causing negative energy. It's negative energy that undermines the determination to get healthy, stay healthy, and do what's right for you.

Achieving a Balance

As clients get rid of their negative energy, I often see their personalities transform. They blossom. They smile more. The twinkle comes back in their eyes. Their posture changes (they stand up a little taller—just short of saluting!). Even the most self-confident and successful people, who have a reputation for being demanding in their work, are often more centered after they've worked with me. I bring out their bright side. Many years ago, I worked with model agency owner Eileen Ford (this was the height of my glitter look—and we were truly the odd couple!), and we had a ball together. One afternoon, we were filming a TV segment with the then Miss Universe (also a client), and something happened to the equipment that required them to reschedule.

Well, the crew was almost shaking in their shoes about breaking the news to Eileen, but she just said, "No problem." The producer, who had done a story about Eileen the previous week and knew that she could be one tough customer, said I must have hypnotized her!

Whoo!

I think my "Whoo!" is my biggest tool for change: my clients and I start off the day that way, and we end it that way (and periodically through the day, if we need a little energy spurt, we let out a Whoo! and our spirits shoot right up).

"Energy Up! Whoo!" snaps people to attention, puts a smile on their faces, and immediately shifts them into a different mode. People stand up taller—they really do! They get sort of sparkly; they move around more when they start unlocking their energy with a Whoo! It's like an electrical jolt, a form of primal therapy—or even being hypnotized in a very positive way!

It's almost impossible not to respond to my Whoo! (it'll wake up the dead, I've been told). When I work with radio stations, I'm constantly Whooing their speakers out! One year, when I did a gig promoting the New York City Marathon, I kept blowing all the systems. They kept saying, "Voltage, lower the Whoo!"

Once I get a client Whooing, I've got 'em, because you can't Whoo! without a smile (sometimes when clients are a little down, they'll call my answering machine knowing I'm not home, just to hear that Whoo! because it energizes them and gives them a lift). And people feel good when they finally do it—they can't help it. Think about when sports fans go to a game: they scream, they yell, they get all psyched up—it's a **RELEASE!** And they feel good because their endorphin levels are being raised.

Sometimes, though, it's the toughest thing to get a client to Whoo! People who are sexually repressed, for example, may have a hard time Whooing. One recent client of mine, a sweetie from one of the wealthiest families in the country, was a little on the uptight side (she didn't find my jokes or stories about sexual escapades amusing in the least; I could see I was going to have to watch my step in order to make a personal connection!). She was also afraid to let go—and she just couldn't Whoo. No way. "That's just not me," she insisted.

When that happens, I just work really hard at pulling it out of them. Usually what I have to do is get 'em into the endorphin state, working out to strong music. Then they'll start Whooing with the music without even realizing what they're doing.

If you're naturally shy, you may also have a hard time Whooing at first (if you think about it too much, you just can't do it!). But a lot of shy people have been taught, "Don't make loud noises, don't do anything that calls attention to yourself, don't rock the boat." Well, I'm saying, "F@#!* that! Rock the boat—and we'll torpedo these negative emotions!" Sooner or later, they all Whoo (once they do, I would venture to say, their behavior in "other areas" may start changing too).

What's Draining Your Batteries?

Because energy blocks turn up in the same basic categories for mostly *everybody,* I've divided them into the following three areas:

Medical

Energy blocks can be caused by a medical condition—which means you need a doctor's checkup to assess what is wrong (there's no way you can feel energized about life when you're in constant physical pain or have a medical condition!). In fact, before I begin working with any client, I strongly recommend he or she get a complete checkup. This goes for you too. Before you start my program, get your doctor's go-ahead. I mean it!

Nutritional

Energy blocks can be nutritional—which is what my eating plan is all about. Many nutritionists and other health experts agree with me that white-flour breads and pastas can be the cause of persistent headaches, grogginess, and what you might call a dragged-out feeling. Sugar gives you that energy rush; then within an hour, it feels like someone's pulled your plug! Salt deadens your taste buds till you can't even taste what you're eating—so you eat more to satisfy yourself—aside from the fact that it's widely believed to contribute to high blood pressure, hypertension, and plain old garden-variety **BLOAT!** Is it just a coincidence that women who suffer from PMS (according to one study, that's fifty to ninety percent of all women, to varying degrees) are advised to give up flour, sugar, salt, alcohol, and caffeine, to help alleviate monthly mood swings, food cravings, headaches, water retention, and breast tenderness? I don't think so!

Many nutritional blocks relate to poor food choices, due to lack of time to eat correctly or lack of knowledge (plenty of otherwise well-informed people just don't realize, for example, how much added sodium there is in the soups, condiments, and breakfast cereals they eat). But frequently, nutritional blocks have an emotional base that has to do with your *relationship* with food—how you use and, possibly, abuse it.

Emotional

Emotional blocks cover relationship issues of all kinds. A problem at work, a love relationship that's getting you down, family conflicts—all affect the way your emotional (or mental) energy manifests itself. Plus, people who are caught up in what others think about them may be horribly blocked—that's a big issue that many clients have. (My own personal motto: *I don't care what anybody else thinks; I care what I think!*).

Now it's time to figure out what's blocking *your* energy. Is it a dead-end job, the prospect of a messy divorce, or a devastating work load with no end in sight? For one of my clients—Risa, a chic brunette in her mid-thirties who just made partner in a **MAJOR** big-city law firm (high-profile, courtroom theatrics were her style)—her energy block was her husband. He was also a big legal eagle, and he sat in with us at our initial interview, belittling her and putting her down about everything.

> **Volt-Note!**
>
> I help clients disconnect from all negative bullshit—and that includes people who don't want you to change. They're looking out for themselves, not you! Keeping you weak (this applies to anything from food and alcohol issues to insecurities about body image and self-esteem) leaves them in control! Once you change from being needy and frightened to being an energy conductor with strength and power of your own, you'll shed people or situations that drain you.

Despite Risa's poise, it was a situation that I could see was ripping her apart inside. When she finally opened up to me, we worked on making her stronger, not just in body, but in mind and spirit. As an energy conductor, I inevitably work on a lot more than food issues! Eventually, her self-worth reached a point where she was strong enough to get rid of anything (and anyone) that wasn't nurturing her—including him!

When I say that I get people to the point where they can do anything they want, I mean it! They're only going to want what *enriches* their lives.

Quiz: Is Your Energy Blocked?

Is your energy blocked? To help you uncover hidden energy blocks, get you to **JUMP YOUR SLUMP** and snap out of it, begin by answering True or False to the following preliminary statement (keep in mind that while there are some days when many of us hate to get up, I am talking about how you feel *almost every day*).

True or False

I hate to get up in the morning.   _____

If your answer is False, more power to you! You probably don't have a **MAJOR** energy block stopping you, which puts you one step closer to getting hooked on the High Voltage lifestyle!

Before you skip to the next chapter, though, remember that even people without *major* energy blocks can still get depressed or experience minor blocks during the day. Some of these could be due simply to lack of sleep. For anyone who's active, sleep isn't a luxury, it's a necessity. Olympic trainers, for example, tell us that enough rest is one of the secrets to stamina! (You have to work your body and then you have to rest your body—because it's when your body is at rest that it replenishes itself. No wonder some days we just feel *tired*.)

Of course, people always assume that I function on very little sleep and are often astounded when they learn that I need a good eight hours—more when I can get it—in order to function. I attribute this to the fact that I usually do more in a day than many people do in a week!

If you answered True to the first statement, then *something* is blocking your energy: something is troubling you that you can't—or don't want to!—face. We need to **IDENTIFY** that energy drain. You have to know what the problem is before you can take steps to change.

First, is it physical? If you haven't had a checkup in the last year, you need to see your doctor. Do it now! Rule out the possibility that your energy drain is due to illness.

Once you've done that, let's examine other possible causes of blockage, which can be anything from money worries and family conflicts to body image and self-awareness.

Part I: Your Working Life   **True or False**

1. On Friday afternoons, when I leave work, I'm so relieved. I thank God that the week is finally over.   _____

2. I love what I do, but I feel like an alien in my office.   _____

3. My boss/supervisor is out to get me and it drives me crazy.   _____

4. I could do my job in my sleep.   _____

5. I always feel like I'm not quite caught up.   _____

6. I'm trapped. I'd leave this job in a minute if I didn't need the money.   _____

7. My job is okay; it's the gossip and the office politics that get me down.   _____

8. My job is going nowhere, but I'm not qualified for anything else.   _____

9. I work alone. My job makes me feel isolated from the whole world. _____

10. I'm in love with one of my co-workers, who is involved with someone else. Now I hate going to the office. _____

If you answered True to any of these statements, obviously your job is a problem that is turning into an energy issue. An on-the-job problem of any kind can deplete your energy, as well as be downright depressing and outright destructive.

If you're not getting satisfaction from your work—the way you spend at least eight hours of every weekday!—the temptation to fall into addictive behavior, whether it's alcohol, drugs, sugar, or other foods, is enormous. These addictions are known for providing the temporary quick fix that gets you past the big, black hole that makes up your daily life.

I don't recommend marching into your boss's office tomorrow and quitting—like most people, you need that paycheck! But you have to deal with why your job is making you unhappy and you have to face the truth. If you don't, you're never going to be able to grow and get past it.

Part II: The Balancing Act   True or False

1. My only moments of "private time" are when I take a shower, get a manicure, or get my hair cut. _____

2. I'm always doing things for everyone else. I never do anything for myself. _____

3. My husband and I haven't had a night alone since the kids were born. _____

4. By the time I get the kids to bed at night, I'm exhausted. _____

5. My mom used to help me out but since she moved away she can't anymore. _____

6. Since my mother died, my father wants to come and live with me. Just when I thought I was free, he can't seem to manage anymore. _____

7. I'm too broke to hire a sitter, so I haven't had a date since my divorce. _____

8. Dating is out of the question for me. As a single mom, I work all day and the only time I see my kids is at night and on weekends. _____

9. My work hours are so long it's not even a question of balancing a personal and a professional life. I don't have a personal life. _____

If you answered True to any of these statements (or if any one of these situations is similar, if not exactly identical, to one in your life), you've identified a major energy blocker.

Sweetie pie, the best thing I can tell you is this: You're not alone. These are problems that are universal. Almost *everyone* today has a little more on their plate than they can handle. But whatever you do about your energy drain, identifying what is causing you to feel overwhelmed—and acknowledging that you have a right to feel that way—is the first step toward finding a creative solution and toward recovery.

For example, if the only time you have alone for yourself is when you get a manicure, then make a religion of it: Get them weekly! Buy yourself some time! If you can't afford to hire extra help with your kids, how about working out a support system with a neighbor or friend with a similar need? (Offer to baby-sit for her kids while she takes an aerobics class, if she'll do the same for you.) Finally, learn to forgive yourself. You are not a bad mother, lover, friend, daughter, or sister if you acknowledge your own need to rest, take a shortcut, or say NO now and then. Often I have to remind a client who feels guilty about taking the time to take care of herself that by doing so, she'll have more energy to take better care of everyone else in her life.

Part III: Relationships

1. Every time I talk to my boyfriend (lover, husband, significant other), I feel like I've put my head in a blender. We both speak English, but we can't communicate. Nothing seems to get through! _____

2. I'm always wondering what my boyfriend (lover, husband, significant other) is really thinking. _____

3. We argue a lot even though we're in love. _____

4. We don't have anything to say to each other anymore—besides talking about the kids. _____

5. My partner and I always do the same things. I'm bored. _____

6. We've been talking about living together, but we never seem to be able to make the decision. _____

7. My true love is married to someone else. _____

8. I can't remember the last time I had great sex . . . or sex at all, for that matter. _____

9. My partner has lost interest in sex. _____

10. Everywhere I go I see happy couples. I'm tired of being alone. _____

11. I haven't had a date (let alone a relationship) in years. _____

12. How could anyone be interested in someone like me? I even turn myself off. _____

If you answered True to any of these statements, realize that problems with relationships can be the biggest drains on your soul and spirit. Once you have true self-love and are whole, however, relationships often become clearer and easier for you to get a handle on, because you're acting from *want, not need.*

Still, the scariest, most energy-depleting thing about relationships is that they're not completely under your own control (and it's often easier to deny that problems exist than to work them out!). But you've taken the first step. Now that you know *what* the problem is, it's time to *talk it out, work it out—or get out. Remember, you truly can't change anyone's behavior. All you can do is change how you respond to it.*

Part IV: **Money**   **True or False**

1. At the end of the month, if it weren't for my overdraft,
    I'd probably be evicted.   _____

2. I pay the minimum requirement on my credit cards each
    month but no more.   _____

3. I'm always short at the end of the week.   _____

4. My husband is working two jobs, and I have to freelance
    to make ends meet.   _____

5. If I leave the house, I don't come home without a
    shopping bag—or two . . .   _____

6. Between school tuition and mortgage payments, I can
    never get ahead.   _____

7. I don't know where my money goes, but it goes. My
    cash seems to fly out of my wallet.   _____

Money is always a biggie! I know it myself: as I always say, being a free spirit can be very expensive these days! Realistically, though, it's not how much money you make—or don't make—that is the issue. It may be a cliché, but money truly doesn't secure happiness (I can attest to that!). When you don't have the financial worries that ninety-nine percent of the people on this planet have, you often make trivial problems much bigger than they really are. To outsiders, it's almost comical—and might be if it weren't so sad.

Money issues can be dealt with. If you worry about money excessively or feel your finances have spun out of control to the point of getting you into *deep trouble,* consult a credit counselor or consider Debtors Anonymous. If your problem is less serious, remember that knowledge is power (you may have to keep a spending diary, just like you keep a food diary). Think of it this way: You may feel like you need another lace bra, but why not wait till the rent check clears?

Part V: Food Issues   True or False

1. If I reach for one cookie, the next time I turn around the bag is empty. _____

2. Every time I have a fight with my boyfriend I turn to the refrigerator. I guess you could say I get my emotional support from Häagen-Dazs. _____

3. In the three months since I broke up with my boyfriend, I've gained ten pounds. _____

4. When I'm really stressed at work, I can't eat . . . and I end up stuffing my face in the middle of the night. _____

5. My schedule is so tight that I can't take the time to eat right. I start my day with a muffin, eat prepackaged soup for lunch—or whatever is handy. _____

6. I've felt like I was fat since I was fourteen.   _____

7. My standby meal is pasta with sauce from a jar. It's fast, easy—and tastes fine.   _____

8. If I eat something I shouldn't, I throw up later or take laxatives.   _____

9. I hate the way I look. I can't stand to look in the mirror.   _____

10. After a long day at work, I usually treat myself to a frozen yogurt. I deserve it.   _____

11. I'd like to get into shape, but I'm too embarrassed to go to an exercise class.   _____

12. I have to keep snack cakes, chips, and treats in the house for my kids—but I end up eating most of them.   _____

13. At work, I just call out for a sandwich and chips for lunch. It's the easiest thing.   _____

14. At least twice a week, I bring home pizza or Chinese take-out food with lots of extra soy sauce from the local restaurant.   _____

15. I eat granola for breakfast, fruit-flavored yogurts and chef's salad with fat-free dressing for lunch. My diet is already healthy.   _____

If you've answered True to one or more of these statements, then your energy block has to do with your relationship with food and your body. This is actually the easiest of the blocks to solve—and we're going to be addressing this directly in the chapters ahead. So read on.

Part VI: Jealousy

1. If my lover leaves me alone in his apartment, I listen to the messages on his answering machine and read his mail.

    _____

2. If one of my friends gets a great new job, I wonder what she's got that I haven't got.

    _____

3. When I go to the beach with my boyfriend, I make sure he doesn't spend too much time helping anyone else put on sunblock.

    _____

4. If I take a friend to a party and she's a big hit with everyone, I don't invite her again.

    _____

5. When I walk down the street and see someone who looks just like I'd like to, I imagine horrible things about her.

    _____

6. If one of my friends tells me that my spouse called her while I was traveling on business, I get really angry at him.

    _____

7. Whenever I see my ex with his stunning new flame, I want to strangle her—or sink under the ground.

    _____

8. I hate shopping with my friends because they can afford nicer clothes than I can.

    _____

9. My ex is dating a woman twenty years younger than I am—she must be a total bimbo.

    _____

10. When my friends tell me about their expensive cars and fabulous vacations, I change the subject.

    _____

11. Whenever my lover talks about his sweetie pie ex, I
    pick a fight. _____

12. I put a phone block on my lover's ex-girlfriend's
    number so she can't call him ever. _____

13. My parents dote on my sister—who is a total screwup.
    Why do I get "penalized" for playing by the rules? _____

14. Whenever my rich friend is looking for a new
    apartment, I can't help but point out the flaws in every
    space she sees. _____

If you answered True to any of the above statements, you have a
problem with jealousy. My dears, you should be crackling with energy down
to your fingertips and you're letting worries about other people block you up!
Jealousy, envy, and good old-fashioned hate zap our energy. Life is too short.
Living with these unreasonable grudges is like walking around with a fifty-
pound sack of sand strapped to your back. What's the point? Let go of your
jealousy and *you* will be lighter. In the end, your life is about you and what
you can do, not about anyone else. Of course, this is easy for me to say (I
have such a short memory I can't remember why someone made me jealous—so I just let it all go!).

I had a beautiful young client, twenty-six, flaming red hair, skin so
creamy it was practically edible, stunning long legs—she was so successful,
so talented, and still she never thought she was pretty enough. She wasted
so much time thinking about what she didn't have, instead of celebrating her
beauty and success. Imagine what a waste that is. She could have been experiencing so much joy.

You have to be thankful for what you have on this planet. If you think
your apartment is too small, look around you at the people who have no
homes. Don't let that ten or fifteen pounds bother you (besides, we can fix
that!). How would you feel if you were sick, or had a terrible accident and
could never walk again?

I beat my young client over the head (that's figuratively, not literally, people!) about how f@#!*ing lucky she was. She had everything in the world going for her. People don't have a clue—what could you be jealous of, really? Love? You have to give it to get it. Money? It just allows you to have a more expensive psychiatrist. It's all the same when you hit the ground, whether you're jumping from a penthouse or a sixth-floor walk-up.

Let's Talk About Sex

Sexuality is an energy block issue that comes up frequently with clients: theirs, somebody else's, whatever, whoever! Now, a sexual dysfunction may be a nonissue for some of you—and that's fine! But if it's not . . .

My basic take on blocks caused by sexual issues is that you should just be honest with yourself—gay, straight, bisexual, whatever—and open with others. The issue that we often have to work out is getting to that personal honesty!

Being open-minded about sexuality is an avenue I use to get closer to people. Many times, sex is a dark, scary issue—and I deal with it with a sense of humor. For example, I play with sexual innuendo all the time. When I host my big music concerts, and come out on stage, saying, "My name is High Voltage and I'm here to help you *get it up . . . your energy up, I mean!*"—I always get a roar of laughter.

Sexual energy blocks can be tricky to deal with. Does a woman have to be in love in order to have sex—and what if she's not in a love relationship at that particular moment? If a marriage is solid all around, *except for the sex,* does this justify having a purely sexual affair, instead of hitting the divorce courts? Should a woman feel guilty about supporting her lover financially—or even paying for sex? (After all, men have been doing this for years!) And what about turning to regular masturbation—as an outlet for sexual tension and energy that is not released in a love relationship? These are all issues that I have had many discussions about with my good friend—and client—best-selling author and radio personality, sex therapist Dr. Judy Kuriansky—and, when the occasion arises with clients, they are issues that I have to deal with too.

Once again, my perspective on sexual energy blocks: Start by being honest with yourself, take the time to define what your own personal moral code is—and move on from there!

Bust That Rut!

Another, even more common energy block I hear about is boredom. People get stuck in a rut and can't think of a way out. Well, get unstuck! Only boring people get bored. But I do hear this frequently and, to be honest, I just don't get it! *I'm* too busy learning new things every day to get stuck on anything!

So jolt your brain. Do something different. Usually we make the mistake of thinking that change has to be something drastic—but that's not always the case. In fact, there are a whole lot of little things (low-cost too!), that you can do to get unstuck—and that can nurture you, mind, body, and soul.

1. **DO** something out of the ordinary. It can be as simple as taking a walk after dinner, joining a new club, or taking up a new activity. The key is to make a **DATE** with yourself and **GET OUT OF THE HOUSE!**

2. **LEARN** something new **(EXERCISE YOUR BRAIN!)**. Take a course. Read a book. Learn a card game. There are so many things to learn and plenty of resources available. Check your local paper and library for postings and information on educational services. And part of the benefit of learning something is that you will meet new people. Need some ideas? For inspiration, turn to page 218, for *123 Things to Do or Think About Instead of Food.*

3. Walk on the **WILD SIDE.** Surprise yourself by doing something unexpected or out of character. If you're a bookworm, give Rollerblading a try. If your last vacation found you lazing on a beach, check out white-water rafting or mountain-biking. If you're into classical music, go to a dance club. See what *other* people are doing for fun!

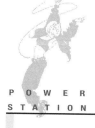

P O W E R
S T A T I O N

STUCK IN

A RUT?

MOVE

YOUR

BUTT!

GET HIGH

ON LIFE,

OR IT'LL

PASS YOU

BY!

4. **PAMPER** yourself. Never had a manicure? Do it now. How about a full-body massage? Go for it! Or get a facial. The key is to realize that you've got absolutely nothing to fear by trying something new. *This planet is loaded with every kind of activity you can imagine.*

THE HIGH VOLTAGE TURN-ON

Stand up straight, lift your shoulders up, back, and down. Come on, do it right now, wherever you are! Up, back, down! Next, I want you to shout: **"ENERGY UP! WHOO!"** Then inhale! Then shout "Whoo!" Let's do this three times together!

Energy Up! (Inhale) Whoo!
Energy Up! (Inhale) Whoo!
Energy Up! (Inhale) Whoo!

Feel the energy! Feel your brain erase the pain! It's that easy! We all have the energy inside of us to change anything we want to, any time of day!

Releasing the Love in Your Heart

Yet another way to dissolve energy blocks is through affirmations—declarations which contain an essential truth that is empowering to you. An affirmation is a phrase or sentence that you repeat to yourself at different times throughout the day. This is a process that can help you reconnect with the universal energy—God, Christ, Buddha, whatever! An affirmation can be as simple as "All is well in my world," or as extensive (and lyrical!) as my own affirmation, below:

Today is a day of completion.
Miracle shall follow miracle,
And wonders shall never cease.

Affirmations are the cornerstones to achieving a High Voltage lifestyle. Don't forget, this is not your standard "diet and exercise" program, it is not just about food—it's about keeping your mind as pure in thought as the food you're putting into your body. We're talking about a life change, from deep within. Without affirmations, while you may lose weight on my program, **YOU WON'T BE ABLE TO FULLY EXPERIENCE THE ENERGY RECHARGE**—which is what this is all about. Remember, High Voltage is a state of mind you can plug in anytime!

For some people, affirmations are just another tool to get a handle on positive thinking. They're a way to reinforce a personal goal, harness your desires and turn them into a new reality. Or, as they would say ("they" being Norman Vincent Peale, Louise Hay, Deepak Chopra, and all the other leading metaphysical messengers), to truly discover your divine design! The best times to do them: when you first wake up in the morning, before you go to sleep at night, and at times of stress or tension during the day (whenever you think you're losing it!). Me personally: I go around humming my affirmations all the time. People who see me on the street think I talk to myself (which in a way, I guess I do). Affirmations can be even stronger when they're done to the beat of music, which is one of the reasons I'm so music-driven. I even do affirmations during my workouts—to my clients' amusement—but the beat of the music only makes them more powerful.

The key to the power of affirmations is to accept that there is some higher power at work that is greater than all of us. It's from this higher, universal power—again, call it what you will—that you get your strength, your energy, your true transformation (this concept, by the way, is the cornerstone of all twelve-step programs from Alcoholics Anonymous to Overeaters Anonymous to Gamblers Anonymous).

Now, if the word "affirmation" sets you on edge, I understand (hey, most of my clients cheer; one, a writer I know, cringed: it's a personal thing!). Different people respond to different messages and messengers. So call them something else—what difference does it make? The point is that for many people—and again, for most of the people I work with—they're effective. Besides, I don't want to get too New Age here—after all, we're entering the **VOLT**-Age, people!

During the time that you're first getting attuned to my program, the right affirmation will eliminate fear, promote inner calm, and help release pent-up, blocked energies that are holding you back. But you need to think out your affirmation carefully. Words are powerful things: there's an old saying, "Be careful what you wish for—you might get it!" (Believe me, I've said that quite a bit to clients.)

Once again, affirmations are deeply personal—at the same time that they reflect a universal truth. What speaks to one person can sound pretentious or trite to another (remember, affirmations don't have to be formal or mystical in tone; they can be as simple or straightforward as you choose). Below, you'll find some personal favorites that I have collected from my clients—who, as you will see from their affirmations, are a varied lot! Use them as a jumping-off point for creating an affirmation that makes life the magical mystery tour it's meant to be. If your affirmation rhymes, it will be easier to remember and to repeat over and over—definitely an advantage when you're doing your aerobic workout to kick-ass music!

P O W E R
S T A T I O N

FREE

YOUR

BODY.

FREE

YOUR

SOUL.

ENER-

GIZE,

TAKE

CONTROL

1. *All is mine by divine design.*
2. *I can do all things through Christ, who strengthens me.*
3. *I am not hungry; I am full and complete; I have everything I need within: life, energy, and love.*
4. *I love and I approve of myself. I see myself and the things I do with eyes of love. I am safe.*
5. *There are no lost opportunities in my divine plan. As one door shuts, another door opens.*
6. *With God, all things are possible.*
7. *Every act committed while angry or resentful brings unhappy reaction.*
8. *What God has done for others, God can now do for me and more.*
9. *The divine plan of my life takes shape in definite concrete experiences that lead to my heart's desire.*
10. *Divine love floods my consciousness with health, and every cell in my body is filled with light.*

If you want to learn more about affirmations, here are some books that have meant a lot to me and had a lot to do with my "transformation": the classic *The Power of Positive Thinking* by Norman Vincent Peale; any book by Louise Hay; and the works of my main girl, Florence Scovel Shinn, who was part of an early-twentieth-century artistic group known as the Eight. Her first book, *The Game of Life,* was written back in 1925 (hey, it's not just me: these ideas have been around a long time!). You'll find four of her best-known works reprinted in *The Writings of Florence Scovel Shinn.* (See Bibliography, page 270)

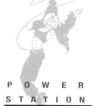

Boost Your Self-Esteem

Other energy blocks have their roots in low self-esteem, which develops when you allow someone else to superimpose their belief system over yours. This happens even to the most high-achieving and creative people. None of us are born with low self-esteem: we are taught to think poorly of ourselves. First it becomes a habit! Then it becomes a reality!

I believe in replacing negative habits with positive ones. The key to learning the habit of positive self-esteem is to bring thoughts of self-love and self-worth into your life's vocabulary. *Now, if you already have a strong sense of self-love and self-knowledge, I don't want to try your patience. Just move right on to the next chapter.* But if you're not there yet, here are three simple "switches" to turn on. If you do them daily, they will become habits that will bring positive change into your life.

Step 1: Change How You Speak

Eliminate phrases from your vocabulary that are disempowering—by that I mean weak, tentative, or wishy-washy. Replace them with strong, positive, life-affirming ones.

> Change "I can't" to "I can."
> Change "I try" to "I will."
> Change "I need" to "I want."

Words are power. Every time you speak, you reinforce your belief in yourself.

Step 2: Hug Yourself

Wrap your arms around yourself and give yourself a big hug. This is important for everyone, but especially if you don't have someone special in your life at this moment—and aren't getting those hugs from anyone else!

No matter how foolish you may feel, hug yourself every morning

P O W E R
S T A T I O N

Put a happy thought in your brain the second you wake up. "I am happy. I am healthy. I have all the energy I need today. Energy Up, Whoo!"

and say: "I love you! I cherish you! I adore you! I want you to be happy!" The point is, you must love yourself before you can love anybody else. People often make the mistake of believing that love has to come to them from the outside, before they can experience transforming emotions.

Well, it's the other way around, folks! You love yourself first; you show your love for others by your positive actions in the world; *then and only then* will love attract itself to you!

Volt-Note!

Mirror, mirror! Can you look in a mirror and say "I love you" and mean it? Can you look in the mirror when you're naked? These are two of the "mirror questions" I ask my clients (who either blush or burst out laughing). Of course, some clients don't even have full-length mirrors, because they would rather not look! One of my clients, an adorable blond ex–cruise director with a sparkling personality, who had put on close to fifty pounds, avoided mirrors like the plague—other than the small mirror she used to put on her makeup. It simply made her too unhappy to face the truth. But you can't change something until you face it. And I don't care what you look like in the mirror—just like I don't care about that number on the scale—because we're going to be changing that. Remember, I'm your number one cheerleader—no matter where you're starting out, it's going to get better! (My darling client—she's thirty pounds down, twenty to go—happens to be my sister Bonnie—and I love her to pieces!)

Step 3: The Mirror Game

This is another way of expressing self-love. Get in front of the mirror and look at yourself—not critically the way so many of us do ("My mouth is crooked," "My thighs are too wiggly"), but with unconditional love . . . and a twinkle in your eye! As I said before, when I look in the mirror I smile and kiss my reflection because I love myself. I don't care how unworthy you might think you are: life is all about loving yourself. It's time to kick self-hate out the door!

In fact, I want you to do it with me right now! Wherever you are, get yourself to a mirror! Dig one out of your purse, grab the rearview mirror in your car, run to the bathroom if you're in your office, whatever—just get in front of a mirror, now.

Now, I want you to look at yourself and say three times **(OUT LOUD)**:

**Mirror, mirror on the wall,
who's the most fabulous one of all?
It's Me! Whoo! It's Me! Whoo! It's Me! Whoo!**

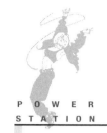

Then, give yourself a kiss.

For some reason (hah!), this simple exercise is difficult for many people. Some people can't even do it AT ALL, at first. But believe me, it's worth getting over that, because it's just so much fun. In fact, when I do this exercise with my clients, it can be very revealing and their responses tell me a lot about what sorts of issues and energy blockers are cluttering up their lives. The only downside: If you get carried away, as I usually do, be sure to have a lot of Windex on hand to get that lipstick off your mirror!

ENERGY UP! WHOO!

P O W E R
S T A T I O N

WE ARE ALL DIVINE BY COSMIC DESIGN! YOU DESERVE HAPPINESS! YOU DESERVE TO BE LOVED! FEEL IT! BELIEVE IT! LIVE IT! ENERGY UP! WHOO!

Chapter 4

ME? I'M NOT A FOOD ADDICT— I CAN CONTROL MY EATING (HAH!)

oes the word "addict" in the title of this chapter scare the hell out of you? Were you even tempted to skip the chapter altogether because you thought the word couldn't **POSSIBLY** apply to you? If so, you're like a lot of people I meet. When I talk about being a food addict, I *know* that the word "addict" is a turnoff. People freak. If there was a better word, I'd use it (in fact, if the phrase "compulsive personality" sits easier with you, **SO BE IT.** Substitute that every time I say "addict"). But whatever you do, give me a chance to explain. Don't close down. Don't immediately shut your mind to the possibility that I could be talking about **YOU.**

It's What Food Means to You

Being a food addict is not a matter of being fat. It is not about lack of willpower or discipline, gluttony, or again, even being tremendously over-weight. You can be a food addict at five four and 127 pounds, dealing with the same ten or fifteen pounds over and over again; you can be stick-thin—anorexic even—or bulimic, or a food addict who's 50 or 60 or 100 pounds overweight. **IT'S ALL THE SAME!**

Being a food addict has to do with your relationship with food—not calories, nor fat content, **but what food means to you, why you want it, and why certain foods make you crazy and make you want more.**

Here are some questions about weight loss that I'm asked frequently:

Q. *Why am I always fighting those same ten, twenty, thirty, or however many pounds?*

A. It's what you're eating, not how much you're eating. Eat what **WORKS** for your body, and the weight will come off and stay off!

Q. *What keeps me from getting to my goal weight, or if I reach my ideal weight on a fad diet, from staying there for any length of time?*

A. A diet filled with addictive substances like flour, sugar, and salt is simply impossible to sustain—and doomed to failure, each and every time.

Q. *When things are bad, isn't it okay, once in a while, to turn to food for comfort—like a midnight quart of ice cream after I've had a fight with my boyfriend?*

A. A binge is a binge: one quart, four quarts, once a month, once every six months. But it doesn't fill the emptiness inside.

If any of the above struck a chord with you, stay with me. *All are indicative of food-addictive behavior.* I'll explain it in the pages ahead.

Being a food addict affects people at different levels. Even if you go on a food binge once a month (and practically starve yourself the next day), even if you feel out of control only periodically, not every day of your life—**you could still be a food addict.**

It's Not in Your Mind

Food addiction (like drug addiction or alcoholism) is an *actual physical addiction*—your body, not your mind, is doing this to you! According to the experts, it's an uncontrollable, real-life craving that is triggered by eating certain addictive foods, even in the smallest amounts (*Betcha can't eat just one*—remember?), and it's usually foods that contain flour, sugar, or salt (a.k.a. processed foods!).

When you are a food addict you cannot touch these addictive foods. Not one morsel!

A lot of people have food addictions and are just not aware of them (they think it's "normal"). If you start with one cookie, is the whole box gone before you realize it? Do you do the same thing with boxes of sweetened cereal, bags of pretzels, or doughnuts? Well, the cycle is caused by something that is actually *in those foods,* and how that something reacts with your body chemistry.

Besides the fact that those three addictive substances—flour, sugar, and salt—bloat you and zap your energy, besides the fact that they are unhealthy (hellooo! **IT'S JUST NOT GOOD FUEL!**), the fact is, there is something in them, sweetie, that triggers addictive behavior—and addictive behavior makes you want more. (Hey, I have spent many years trying to disprove my theory and when I finally faced the truth, it was a relief beyond belief. I wanted to scream it from the rooftops—which in my own way, I guess, I'm doing all the time!)

If you're a food addict, you can't stop eating whatever it is that you're addicted to, and a lot is never enough. Many food addicts, fat or thin, wake up thinking about food, go to sleep thinking about food, and in between are figuring out what, where, and how much they are going to eat! Do you want to know how I can really tell when somebody may have a food addiction? If they get almost angry when I say they can't have white flour. "I can't live like that, I can't," they yell. They respond so strongly that it's almost violent!

Believe me, it's amazing how much energy goes into this kind of behavior. If you could take that energy and do something constructive with it, you could probably build a world-class career! (Don't I know it: it takes as much energy to be f@#!*ed up as it takes to function well!) If you have a tremendous natural energy level, that energy, used the wrong way, can destroy you! Until you redirect it, it can be a **BIG BAD MONSTER!**

Come Clean with Yourself

Maybe you don't think you're a food addict. Or maybe you're just not sure. One client of mine, a well-known Seventh Avenue fashion designer who now looks as trim as one of her own models, originally couldn't see herself as an addict at all: she wasn't terribly overweight, didn't have a house full of junk food, never went on food binges—or so she protested. But people's food addictions are manifested in different ways. Remember, a food addiction has to do with your *relationship* with food and what that food does to you, and your feelings about how, why, and what you eat. If you eat because of stress or when you're tired, or to "reward" yourself, you're treading perilously close to food addict territory, whether you admit it or not.

Another client, Damien, thirty, a recovering alcoholic and drug addict (and now, an admitted food addict), is another example. "I never kept alcohol, dope, or even much food in the house, but I'm an addict just the same," he explains. "I just pursued my addictions on the outside!"

If you're not sure if you are a food addict or have addictive tendencies (if you were brought up in this country, I could almost guarantee that you do!), ask yourself the questions in the checklist that follows:

The Food Addict's Checklist

1. If you stuff your face at your best friend's birthday party—you just couldn't leave that cake alone—do you empty yourself afterwards by vomiting or taking laxatives?

2. Are you a human yo-yo, always "sort of" on a diet, losing the same ten pounds and gaining them back over and over?

3. Do you spend half your workday thinking about what you're going to eat when you get home?

4. When you go down a size, is it like a shot of happiness?

5. Do you have a secret stash of your favorite food so your spouse or kids can't find it and eat it?

6. Once you've had "just a taste" of bread, bagels or muffins, crackers, pasta, salty snacks, or sweets, can you stop? Or do you keep going back for "one more"?

7. Do you think about food or your weight night and day? Or about your next diet?

8. Would you be embarrassed if your best friend really knew everything you ate yesterday? Would you be ashamed to keep a food diary—a truthful one—and share it with your spouse or lover?

9. Do you sneak food on the sly?

10. Do you eat healthily when other people are around, but lose it completely when you're alone?

11. Once you start to snack, do you find it impossible to stop?

12. When you want to lose weight, is it easier for you to skip meals altogether rather than just eating smaller ones?

13. Do you often feel tired or "wiped out" after a meal?

14. Are you tired all the time? Are there things that you'd love to do, but you just don't have the energy?

15. Are you hungry again two hours after you eat? If you have a big meal—even with dessert—do you want another just a few hours later?

16. Do your moods swing from high to low? Are you lonely? Depressed?

If you've answered "yes" to any of the odd numbers, you are probably a food addict. Discovering this can be freeing for many of us (for one thing, you know it's not your "fault"). What we're going to do is to set up a formula that allows you to eat in a healthy way and that stays away from the substances that trigger your addictive behavior. And believe me, once you've taken them out of your diet, you'll be so grateful and so thankful that you have more time and more energy to spend on the real issues of your life, that you just won't want them back anymore.

If you've answered "yes" to more than two of the even numbers, you may not be an out-and-out addict, but you may have food-addictive tendencies that are being triggered by flour, sugar, or salt.

Recognize Your Addiction

So, are you a food addict? I am—and so are many of my clients, and a lot of the people I know (maybe that's why they're drawn to me!). I think that a lot of very creative and talented and fabulous people are prone to addictive behavior (often it's the other side of the coin from all that talent and energy!).

Of course, I have an addictive personality, period. I know it—and I accept that that's who I am. I can't drink and I don't drink (if I did, I'd wake up with strangers!). Every once in a while, I used to think it might be fun to have a glass of champagne—but I can't have that glass, just like I can't have a slice of cake or pizza, because then I'd eat the whole cake—or fifteen pizzas!—and become bulimic again.

I can't do "a little bit" of this and "a little bit" of that. I know because I've tried to, over and over again. And you know what? I can't and neither can millions of other people either!

But the good news: I don't even want to anymore—thank you very much!

Frequently people who are prone to food addictions are susceptible to eating disorders like anorexia, bulimia (to help control their food addiction!), and compulsive eating or to addictive behavior in general—like drugs, smoking, or alcohol abuse. I'm a prime example of that! After I kicked drugs, which kept me skinny (cocaine acts as an appetite suppressant, heroin keeps you thin because you're just too f@#!*ed up to eat, which is why it's rampant in the fashion industry!), I became bulimic in order not to become fat. I was literally throwing up all the time in the early and mid 1970s. It wasn't until years later that my teeth started to rot (those juices in the stomach are like acid—powerful stuff!). To this day, my periodontist is one of my best friends!

Just as often, food addiction is an isolated condition. *You may never have taken up smoking, you may never have gotten into drugs, you may have no problem with alcohol, you may not even have much of a weight problem.* Again, it may only be ten or fifteen pounds that you're struggling with (that you either can't drop or that you've lost and regained over and over again), *all because you are sensitive to the addictive effects of flour, sugar, and salt.*

The thing you really need to know **FOR CERTAIN** is that food addictions are **REAL. BELIEVE IT!** I can't stress this strongly enough. Think about it. If you eat pasta or bread or chips, do you seem to eat more than you intended? Hey, do you ever see people bingeing on lettuce? Or not being able to control their fruit salad?

But even though we've known about food addictions for over fifty years (I didn't discover this and I'm not making it up), food addiction is still not considered a "legitimate" addiction by the general public.

What do I mean? Well, most people these days acknowledge that *alcoholism* is a true addiction. When was the last time you heard someone urging a recovering alcoholic to have "just a sip, it won't hurt you" of champagne, a martini, or Scotch on the rocks? *It's just not done.* Yet, when it comes to food, somehow we're still in the Stone Age: people are **ALWAYS** saying, "How can one little taste hurt? You have willpower, don't you?"

Hellooo! Willpower is **NOT** *the issue.*

My approach to food addiction is that if you are going to cut flour out of your diet, look at flour as if you're an alcoholic and know that first bite of a dinner roll, forkful of fettucine, or nibble of French toast is the same as an alcoholic's sipping a glass of wine. It's the same principle, people! Not long ago, I had dinner at Elaine's, a popular Manhattan bistro, with an incredibly successful theatrical publicist who happened to be a client, plus two business associates who weren't. My client, Richard, who had lost twenty-three pounds working with me over the past three months (and had maybe ten or twelve pounds more to go), reached for the basket of flatbread in the middle of the table and said, "Oh, I'll just break off a little piece." And our "well-meaning" companions agreed that "just a taste" couldn't possibly do Richard any harm.

I am so glad I was there. Of course, as I do with all my clients, I had explained my alcohol analogy to him earlier. But Richard was a fairly new client and the Voltage ways were not second nature to him. Fortunately, I knew just what buttons to push to get him back in line. "Sweetie, while you're at it, why don't you just have a glass of wine too?" I asked him. There was dead silence at the table, as he put the cracker down—because he knew exactly what I meant—and I called for the waiter to have the bread basket removed. Abstinence means abstinence, guys—you can't do it halfway!

Richard, by the way, was incredibly relieved to discover he was a food addict. In fact, his relief bordered on absolute elation! Here, at last, was a reasonable explanation for what he had been going through. His food addiction was as powerful as an alcohol addiction. One bite would have led to two . . . which would have led to buying and eating a bag of pretzels, then all the other flour products he could get his hands on . . . and eventually to his regaining the twenty-three pounds—and then some!

Even though I had been pounding my philosophy into Richard's

The fact is, when you're an addict ***you're an addict.*** *Until you* **wake up** *and f@#!*ing* **deal** *with that, you're going to be on a yo-yo, up and down all the rest of your life.*

71

brain since our initial meeting, like many of us in social situations, he simply went on automatic pilot and, without my verbal cue, was about to revert to his old patterns.

Eventually, the message takes. As I said before, when we're changing the tapes in your brain, we have to do it over and over and over again, until the connection sticks (there's no magic here, sweetie pies!). So if I go on and on about certain subjects—yes, you have heard it before. And trust me, you will again, until I get through! I get big bucks for beating people over the head with this, and I'm doing this book for **YOU!**

Volt-Note!

By the way, let me point out that being a food addict doesn't mean you're always out of control or stuffing yourself. It does mean that you need to acquire a lifestyle where you're not always focused on food, and one that gets your body in the best shape possible (like living at a spa—which is why I loved it so!).

Plus, food addiction has nothing to do with enjoying the taste of certain foods—just as alcoholism is not about enjoying the taste of Scotch or vodka or whatever. Just as you learn to love the taste of alcohol, you can learn to love the tastes of different foods. And in addition to getting you to love different things, my job is also to separate you from your attachments to food. I don't want food to be your joy. I don't want food to be your best friend. I don't want food to be how you reward yourself (all too common in our society!). Finally, just remember that even if you don't have an out-of-control food compulsion, sooner or later it could easily become one. Nothing starts out full-blown, nothing.

Know What Sets You Off

Some food addicts are prone to bingeing and purging to help "control" their addiction. Others hoard food. Others exercise like maniacs, while some fool themselves by filling up on foods they consider healthy or "nonfattening."

One client of mine, Lisa, a screenwriter, remembered that years ago, as a college freshman in Virginia, she had binged on boxes of granola cereal (remember Quaker Oats "Natural" cereal in the big yellow box—one of the first commercial granolas in the 1970s? I sure do!). Whenever Lisa poured a bowl, she just kept going back for another, and another, till the whole box was gone! And even though "Natural," of course, implied that the cereal was healthy, the reality was **BIG-TIME** calories and sugar—which meant big trouble for all those food addicts out there, me included!

Now, I'm not a big fan of many breakfast cereals—besides oatmeal, rolled oats, cream of rice, and a few others—but the fact is, granola cereals often are coated with sugar and oil to glue the crunchy oats together. That means you don't get more vitamins or fiber; you do get a whole lot more calories and fat!

I've also had clients who planned tours and vacations strictly around food—often to their tremendous inconvenience! One client from San Francisco even rerouted a European flight plan so he would have a layover in a specific country—with just enough time for him to drive from the airport to a famous bakery so he could taste their cream-filled pastry! Now that's a serious problem!

Other times, the addiction is more subtle. One of my clients, a pretty champagne blonde and a major player on the New York charity circuit, felt she had to keep peanut butter in the house for her two young children, and counted on her nanny to hide the jar (if she didn't see it, she wouldn't want it). But if she found it (and she sometimes searched the cabinets high and low in the middle of the night), she'd eat it all at one sitting. I switched her to a salt-and-sugar-free brand, which eliminated the addictive physical craving. And by the way, her kids got used to the healthier peanut butter in no time—they didn't even notice the change!

Another client, also a prominent socialite, with an enormous Park Avenue apartment, requested that her husband put a special lock on the refrigerator door at night. Dead-bolting the fridge was the only way to stop her midnight raids, she told me. This only worked because it was at her request (the couple was working together as a team on her problem). Mind, this sort of behavior is not unusual for food addicts. It happens a lot until they get a handle on their addictions—which, in the case of this client, we eventually did.

We're All Raised to Have Food Addictions!

Of course, I'm not the only one who was brought up on food like this. We all were! In this country, people are practically raised to have addictions: I always say if you've been given flour and sugar since you were a baby, you start off wacky! Think about those so-called "terrible twos" that toddlers go through. Ever think it's because the poor kids are in sugar shock half the time? Waffles with syrup, sugary cereals, sweetened baby food—ugghhh! *Our parents didn't know any better, but we do.* Clients of mine who have children and don't feed them any sugar tell me their little darlings never go through that two-year-old nightmare stage. Now I don't think that's a coincidence, do you?

What Do I Feed My Kids?

Sometimes people ask me how they should feed their children. Well, how about the same healthy, High Voltage way that *you're* learning to eat! Kids don't need Cheez Doodles and M&M's! Do you love your kids? Do you want them to be healthy? Then why do they need sugar and garbage food? If sugar were a drug, you wouldn't dream of giving it to your kids.

I had one client who came from a family with serious weight disorders. It hadn't manifested itself in her as much as it had in other family members, and in particular, one child, a boy of twelve, who was about fifty or sixty pounds overweight! My client wanted me to work with her son (even more than with her), but I said no. "Let's get you to change your lifestyle, and your family will follow," I suggested. "You can't tell your child, 'Don't eat bread,' if *you're* still eating it! The best example is when you do it yourself, and then it becomes the family way of doing things!"

That's why, when I work with clients, I like the whole family to get involved. And they often do. Once other family members see the client feeling better, looking better—and healthier—they all want to do the same thing. Besides, "Do as I say, not as I do" never works!

So back to the question—what do you feed the kids? Well, the same things you're going to be eating yourself: all the delicious, fresh, back-to-nature foods from our planet. Wholesome oatmeal. Eggs. Juicy grapes, oranges, pears, berries, and other fruits. Calcium-rich yogurt (with sliced strawberries and bananas on top, it's like a healthy ice cream sundae!). Sliced breast of turkey, with carrots and sweet potatoes (kids love those orange veggies). You get the idea. Get creative!

How Food Addicts Get Hooked

Having a food addiction can be a vicious cycle. Many food addicts—through tremendous willpower, I might add!—manage to diet strenuously for a few weeks or months, and lose weight—only to see the compulsion take hold and the diet fail, and to regain the weight they lost (and then some).

Food addicts often try diet after diet—from liquid diets to fasting to stomach stapling!—in an effort to control their addiction. Even "sensible" diets, which counsel moderation, are not always the solution! For some of us—possibly you too?—even a tiny little bit of any of those lethal, addictive substances will set you off! **The only permanent solution is to recognize the addiction and to eliminate completely from your daily diet those foods that are causing it.** Period. End of story.

Often people are food addicts without even knowing it. I never knew. When I was with my husband and he was eating huge meals, I joined him, course after course after course—only I would throw up in between each one (in those days, I would buy a Sara Lee pound cake and eat the whole thing at one sitting—and I never even focused on the fact that it had become a compulsion).

I wasn't the only one doing it either. *I* learned my wonderful new system at Saratoga from the jockeys and their wives, who also taught me the sitting-in-the-sauna-wrapped-in-cellophane trick (their sure-fire way to drop two to three pounds of water weight fast).

Water Pills—an Addictive Crutch

Some women who are compulsive about their weight get addicted to water pills—it's a fast way to drop as much as three pounds overnight, and another trick I learned at Saratoga, from one of the world's most famous jockeys, when I was just twenty-five and my husband and I used to go there for the races (in those days I would get addicted to anything!). Jockeys, of course, are fanatic about weight—any extra pounds and they get fined! Well, I took one of the pills he gave me—Lasix, a very powerful water pill—and, bang, three pounds were gone. Soon, water pills became my crutch. I was constantly popping them—to look better in a bare little dress or a special evening gown. And they can be a nightmare, people! They'll take you to a certain point, but they also hurt your kidneys, possibly increase your cholesterol levels (although who knew about this or cared back then!), and get you so weak you'll pass out. Years later, I also saw many of the supermodels popping water pills, especially when it was period time and they had to be on that runway.

Now, there may be times when a water pill is necessary (talk with your doctor), but don't become dependent on them. Of course, I found a natural way of eliminating excess water weight by taking salt out of the diet (a whole lot healthier than pill popping). Take the salt out of your diet, girls, or at least cut down, and even if you normally blow up five pounds like clockwork when you get your period, I guarantee it won't be as much. Plus, eliminating water by natural means is a much safer way to go, so look into natural diuretics, like taking vitamin B_6, drinking corn silk tea (or any of the many other "slimming" herbal or PMS-formula teas), even eating asparagus!

Evolution of a Food Addict

Today, while my addictions are rechanneled (I'm now addicted to energy!), one thing I want to make clear is that **I am as addictive today as I have ever been.** If you have an addictive personality, that will never change. All you can do is change the destructive addiction to a positive one—like exercise, or a job you love—that makes your life work.

Looking back at how I was raised, it's not so hard to see how my eating patterns evolved: I've always had a tendency to go for the floury, starchy stuff. Back in the small town in Ohio where I grew up (in an Italian household with a mother who loved to cook!), I practically lived on pasta dishes like lasagna and ravioli. Plus, throughout my childhood, I was attracted to dough—pie dough, cookie dough, pancake batter, you name it. Now that may seem normal enough to you (most kids like doughy sweets), but it's not normal when you're compelled to keep going back for more and more and more!

Now, I was so active as a kid—I was a figure skater and a dancer—that all this eating didn't really show up in my weight . . . although looking back at myself in high school—at five four and 135 pounds—by today's standards, no doubt about it, I was a little chunky! I still have my high school graduation picture and my face is as round as an apple! But remember, this was the tail end of the Marilyn Monroe and Jayne Mansfield era: well-padded curves were sexy. Back then, we girls wanted to make our hips bigger, not smaller! (Now, I'm five four and 104 pounds—I like being a little underweight!)

In my family (whom I love dearly!), how-ever, obesity was the norm. Compared to every-one else, I was thin! But I broke the cycle. You can too. *Remember, I am probably the best proof that no matter how screwed up and dysfunctional you've been, you can not only make your life work, you can thrive—and enjoy it!*

Why You **Can't "Just Say No"**

For you hard-core food junkies out there (do you like this word better?) who see yourselves in the addictive behavior I've described, a serious food addiction can be more difficult to kick, in some ways, than a drug or alcohol addiction. Let me explain why.

> ## Volt-Note!
> When the Twiggy era dawned, I left home, and dis-covered methamphetamines, commonly referred to as speed (one of the "great" side effects of the drug was that you couldn't eat—which is why so many eating disorders are disguised when you're into drugs). Cocaine also enabled me—and all the mod-els I hung out with—to stay thin. (Don't kid your-self—if you're not naturally thin, drugs are the only way anyone can possibly stay that thin!) Some of my clients—major models—didn't even realize that they had food addictions until they had dealt with their drug addictions. Afterwards, when they blew up like balloons (their weight, I mean!), they had to relearn their eating patterns all over again. One very famous face had to leave the business entirely.

Eventually, after a weaning-off period, you have to go "cold turkey" on drugs; you give up drugs and/or alcohol *com-pletely* (I'm a strong advocate of the effectiveness of all those twelve-step programs). But you can't go cold turkey on food! *You have to eat to live; you have to confront food—and make healthy choices—every single day of your life. Putting it plainly, if you're an alcoholic, you don't drink. But if you're a food addict, you still have to eat.*

Forget About Just One Bite

As I said before, most people are much more understanding about alcohol or drugs than they are about food addiction, and are more willing to acknowledge that the addiction is **REAL.**

But as someone who has struggled to kick a drug addiction, *and* as a recovering alcoholic, I have no problem with the idea of food addiction. In fact, as with my client Richard, the theatrical publicist, discovering that one's food addictions are real can actually be a relief to many people, especially if they've been trying to lose weight for years and can't, or if they've tried dozens of diets, only to lose weight at first and then see the pounds creep back on.

But some of you might be *more comfortable* with the idea of thinking of your addiction as a violent and serious *allergy*—one where just a taste of a potentially addictive food (such as an ice cream cone, salty potato chips, or even one of those fat-free-but-loaded-with-sugar-and-calories muffins) can set off a bout of uncontrollable bingeing. One client of mine, Brett, thirty-four, a dashing southern real estate mogul, whose charm would melt your heart, fell off the wagon with salty french fries—stealing one, then another and another from his dinner partner's plate, until he finally polished off the entire plate. Then he ordered a basket of his own—and one to go!

For those of you who, like Brett, fall into this category, it's probably far easier for you to swear off pasta or bread entirely than to eat a small, "sensible" amount. "I'd rather forget about cheesecake entirely than have just a sliver," one of my clients, a brilliant (and busy!) interior designer—and real sweetie pie—confessed to me. (I understood completely! Cheesecake was once my favorite too!) But I know now—as does my client—that it takes only one forkful to trigger a craving, which leads to taking one bite after another, till the whole sinful slice is gone (and for New York–style cheesecake, that's about 800 calories for a single slice!). I tell her just what I tell all my food addict clients: "Take it one day at a time!" It's a phrase that you'll hear in all addictive programs.

Falling Off the Wagon

People like my client the interior designer and reformed cheesecake fan are the reasons why I can't emphasize strongly enough the pitfalls of taking that first "little bite"—during the first days of my program and especially after you've been at it for a few months and getting results. The usual thinking in this last instance is, "I'm doing so well, looking so good, how could one bite hurt?"

But if you're a hard-core food addict, I guarantee that if you take that first bite you'll be in trouble again. It's like a ball rolling downhill. **PLEASE, DON'T HAVE SUCH A SHORT MEMORY FOR YOUR PAIN, MY FRIENDS! DON'T FORGET WHAT THESE FOODS DO TO YOU!**

Backsliding can be traumatizing. I've been on the phone with clients for hours sometimes, reinforcing my message. But in the end, you just have to start all over (again, I believe in taking it one day at a time). Probably one of the most important things is not to set yourself up for ultimate failure by using backsliding as an excuse to go backward permanently. I don't let my clients do that, and I'm not going to let you do that!

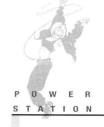

P O W E R
S T A T I O N

Think of it this way: Once you start my program, day by day, it's like building a wall, brick by brick. Eventually you're going to have a very strong wall—one that is able to stand up to people (some well-meaning, **MANY NOT**) who urge you to eat or drink things that you know are lethally addictive and destructive to your body, your energy, your ultimate happiness, and your life!

And hey, sometimes even I let my guard down—although never with flour. Flour is my f@#!*ing enemy and I know it. I look at it and I just see cellulite in every form! But every once in while, in a restaurant, I'll be served something that tastes a little salty—even though I've specified no salt—and I'll eat it anyway. When that happens, I can usually count on waking up the next day with puffy hands and feet and not feeling all that well. After a while, I tell you, it's just not worth it. I love being energetic. I love being vivacious. I won't allow anything to take that away from me.

DON'T LET A TASTE THAT LASTS JUST A SECOND RUIN THE NEW LIFE YOU ARE BUILDING FOR THE FUTURE.

With Me, What You See Is What You Get!

I don't generally attack people's eating habits in restaurants, although I do ask that the salt shaker and the bread basket be removed from the table (I find it disrespectful of who I am and what I stand for). And when I see people eating linguine with marinara sauce or spaghetti carbonara, I don't ever think, Oh, I wish I could eat that but I know I can't. I think, Schmuck! Bigtime! To me, pasta is just a plate of cellulite with sauce on top!

A Healthy Choice

Someone once asked me how I handle things when I'm out for a social evening and don't want to make other people uncomfortable. But the fact is—I do want to make people uncomfortable! I am who I am: I don't change into something else when I get home. If you invite me, it comes with the package. (Hey, if you're embarrassed to eat dinner with me, that only tells me that you must feel there's something wrong with your eating habits, hmmmm.) Besides, remember that not only do most people **WANT** to have me around, they **PAY** to have me around! (But I admit it: I don't get invited out to many dinner parties unless they're mine—and I'm controlling the food!)

What If You're Not a Food Addict?

Now some of you may not be food addicts, but you may have addictive tendencies. I think of it

> #### ∼ Volt-Note! ∼
>
> **B**ecause I spent so many years as a bulimic, eating huge amounts of food, I am hypercareful. To this day, I could never cut myself a single slice of cake (I would eat the whole cake!) or sample a single cookie (it would be more like three dozen!). That's why bulimia seemed logical to me—there was no way I could keep all that in my stomach!
>
> So this way—the **HIGH VOLTAGE** way— is easier; the other way—totally wanting, totally compulsive—was a painful nightmare, and not a place that I, or **ANYONE**, would want to live psychologically! If you're the same way, I say, give it up! What's so hard about it? What the hell are you losing—torture? The right to wear a size 18? You can get addictive foods out of your system, just as others get drugs out of their systems!
>
> If you can experience what it's like to be in control and go on with your life—to know that every thought shouldn't be about food—then it's worth a shot. **NO FLOUR, NO SUGAR, NO SALT**— this is not a scary way to live; this can be salvation! Believe me, it's the other way of life—the food addict's way of life—that's truly dark and frightening!

as being just *mildly compulsive.* If that's you, if you are not a food addict but are still **SENSITIVE** to certain foods, *you will still feel better, look better, and have a higher, healthier energy level when you follow an eating plan that steers clear of the addictive foods to which your body reacts.*

Finally, if you're the rare bird who is not food-sensitive at all, and you are simply looking to boost your energy level (maybe even lose a few pounds in the bargain?) and find a healthier way of living and eating that will serve your body (and the planet!) better in the long run, **ENERGY UP!** will benefit you too!

One Giant Step Ahead of the Scientists (or Why Me? What's to Blame?)

Many people ask me what causes addictive foods to be addictive to some people and not others—and it's a good question! Is it genes? Hormones? Some chemical in the brain? The fact is, there are many different schools of thought floating around out there right now, which all add up to this: **WE JUST DON'T KNOW!**

I've listened to all the theories, read the books, and I've actually debated with myself (and my editors!) as to whether or not I should call in a doctor to explain how addictions physically work. But the problem is that the doctors can't even agree among themselves!

Now, I'm not a doctor or a research scientist and I don't go in for a lot of pseudoscientific jargon, fancy percentages, complicated charts and formulas. People eat food, not formulas! I do go for common sense. So here's my take on it.

Personally, I don't care who is right or who is wrong. In fact, I choose not to enter the debate. But I do know that some of you might need the reassurance that plenty of respected medical doctors have also identified the addictive characteristics of flour, sugar, and salt, and are studying and documenting it—and they are!

But until the day when they all agree **(DON'T HOLD YOUR BREATH, PEOPLE)**, you're going to have to make a leap of faith here and rely on what I have seen prove itself over and over again: My personal experience as an addict, and my practical experience with others, has shown me over and over that this "theory" is stone-cold fact! **FLOUR. SUGAR. SALT.** These three white powders **ARE** triggers, my friends. **WHY THEY ARE TRIGGERS IS JUST NOT AS IMPORTANT AS RECOGNIZING THE FACT THAT THEY ARE.** (Remember that while no one has proven exactly what causes alcoholism, you'd be hard-pressed to find anyone who would dispute the fact that it exists!)

> **Volt-Note!**
>
> I know, I know. You can find statistics to suit any purpose. Still, I can't resist telling you that the American Heart Association agrees with me that there are no quick fixes! Any diet based on a single food (like the popular cabbage soup diet) or on combining two foods (beets and peanut butter!—no kidding!) in order to burn fat, is **TOTAL NONSENSE!** In fact, they've come out in favor of a diet that's low in fat, high in fruits and vegetables—which is exactly what I've talked about for years!

I have to admit that I do get a chuckle out of seeing science catch up with me—as it has lately, **BIG-TIME!** All of a sudden we're reading about what I've known and told my clients for years: that flour—in pasta, in bread, in bagels and cake and doughnuts—makes people fat. **BIG SURPRISE!**

In fact, we're starting to see articles about the addictive qualities of flour **EVERYWHERE!** "Banish the bagel." "Are you a carb addict?" "Wear Italian, don't eat Italian." It's even touted as the "diet secret" of many of the stars!

Some food experts have come out against carbohydrates; still others promote food combos or even certain combinations of medications. Richard and Rachael Heller of New York's Mount Sinai Hospital, for instance, are a well-known physician and nutritional researcher who have written extensively about carbohydrate addictions. They say that nearly seventy-five percent of all overweight people are probably carbohydrate addicts—pretty devastating in a world that is shoving pasta, croissants, and bagels down your throat at every corner restaurant! Then there's *The Zone*, of course, by Barry Sears, Ph.D., who flat out condemns carbs. Throw out pasta, rice, bread, and grains, he writes, for lasting fat loss, great health, and peak performance. I could go on and on . . . *but just keep in mind that all of these experts and their theories have both their supporters and detractors.*

What do I think? Listen: I've been around long enough to watch everything come and go, and come and go—*and I'll still stick with my Ph.D.*

in common sense and my diploma from the University of the Streets (I may shop on Madison Avenue, but I don't *listen* to Madison Avenue!). And my common sense tells me (and yours should too!) that when you eat **PASTA,** when you eat **CAKE,** when you eat **BREAD** and **FRENCH-FRIED POTATOES, CHOCOLATE-GLAZED DOUGHNUTS** and **CHEETOS**—you get fat. Period. You don't need a five-year government grant, a ten-year study, and a string of letters after your name to tell you that!

Food (Addiction) for Thought

If my quiz about food addiction has struck a chord, or if you think you may be sensitive to (if not outright addicted to) flour, sugar, and salt, you may want to read further about the insulin connection and seratonin (it's a brain chemical), both of which have been linked to food addictions, and about compulsive eating disorders, and see what the "experts" are saying. (Just remember, they seldom all agree!)

One terrific book that explores food addictions in general in a thoughtful and compassionate way is Kay Sheppard's *Food Addiction: The Body Knows.* "Food addiction is chronic, progressive and ultimately fatal," she writes. And the Hellers talk directly to carb addicts in their many works; one to check out is *The Carbohydrate Addict's Diet.*

But if you don't choose to look further, trust me, it's not something you need to do for the purposes of understanding my program!

Also, if you're still uncomfortable with the word "addict," call your need whatever you want! I call it a relief—for me and many others—just to know it exists. And hey, my program will work for you anyway, squeamish about the word "addict" or not (trust me on that one too).

Tune in to My Program

The program that I am going to outline for you in the chapters ahead is equally as beneficial and empowering to the food addict, the nonaddict, or the person somewhere in between. Flour and sugar and salt are not good for

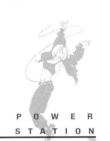

ANY BODY. Even if they don't affect you in a way that triggers addictions (which, frankly, would be hard for me to believe!), these foods are still basically valueless when it comes to a healthy, high-voltage lifestyle.

If you're a food addict, or if you have addictive tendencies, you have to live and eat this way in order to function **AT YOUR BEST** in this world.

If you are not prone to food addictions but simply want to take off a few pounds, **KEEP THEM OFF, HAVE MORE ENERGY, FEEL BETTER, AND PUT THAT TWINKLE BACK IN YOUR EYE, IT WILL WORK FOR YOU TOO.**

The First Day of the Rest of Your Life

My clients usually start off with **SPA WEEK,** a seven-day jump-start program in which we introduce my **STAR POWER PLAN** and strictly eliminate flour, sugar, and salt. This allows you to lose your taste and compulsion for these addictive substances—and get them **OUT OF YOUR SYSTEM.** Just as in alcohol or drug addiction, you need to dry out!

During **SPA WEEK,** as your body is cleansing and adjusting, you may be uncomfortable for a few days—sometimes (not always) people get headaches, are grouchy, lethargic, or even dizzy. These "withdrawal symptoms" usually pass after several days (how long depends on you: if you're a heavy junk food junkie, your withdrawal may last longer).

It's especially important during this time not to give in to your food cravings, which is why I like to be with my clients 24/7 during their **SPA WEEKS** . . . and why you might do well to consider doing my program with a friend for support (the buddy system always works!).

Usually by the end of the first week you'll see—and feel—a change. You actually start to not want these things (and after a period of time, your resolve will increase). As you see your body changing—and energies recharging—flour, sugar, and salt become the enemies! Remember, this is war!

So, are you ready to let go of the fat-producing, energy-depleting, mind-depressing, **ADDICTIVE** foods packed with **FLOUR, SUGAR, AND SALT** that are controlling your life? Like ice cream. Or burritos. Or especially pizza. Now there's a food addict's nightmare! It's doughy bread, salty cheese, sugared-up sauce (commercial tomato sauces are loaded with sugar and salt), even when it's not topped with fatty, salty, artery-clogging sausages or pepperoni (mmmmm . . . I don't **THINK** so!). People often ask me if my program is guaranteed to work. Well, if you're really looking for a guarantee, keep eating the way you have been. It's practically guaranteed to make you tired, make you sluggish, and make you fat!

So are we ready to get back to common sense? Are we all clear that this is not about willpower, that this is not about discipline? (Dieters are the most disciplined people of all. My God, they're **ALWAYS** dieting). Then turn to the next chapter, take a look at my **STAR POWER PLAN,** and let's declare WAR against those three white powders together!

ENERGY UP! WHOO!

Chapter 5

STAR POWER!
NO FLOUR,
NO SUGAR,
NO SALT,
NO KIDDING!

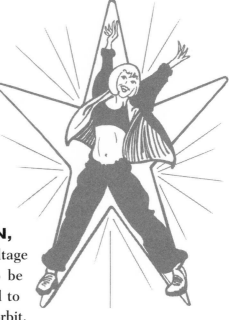

The cosmic core of my program is my **STAR POWER PLAN,** which contains the Ten High Voltage Commandments. This is going to be your guiding **STAR**—all you need to know to get yourself in the right orbit.

On one side of the star, you'll find the first five power points: no flour, no sugar, no salt, avoid processed foods, and drink plenty of water. On the flip side of the star you'll find the next five—the categories of fresh, beautiful foods that are going to give you **STAR POWER,** and make your energy soar: fruits and vegetables; grains; chicken, fish, and meats; healthy fats; and low-fat, no-salt dairy products.

Danger! High Voltage!

Let me begin with the nuts and bolts: those three addictive substances—flour, sugar, and salt—which I've already identified in the previous pages. Eliminating these three white powders from your diet is nonnegotiable—and by now you should know I mean it! No ifs, ands, or buts! In fact, if it helps, when you see something with flour in it, or with salt, or when you're about to reach for a sugary cookie or other snack, I want you to hear bells going off in your head!—**DANGER! HIGH VOLTAGE!** And stay away!

If I haven't convinced you yet about their addictive, doom-your-diet powers, ask yourself the following questions: Is the way you're eating now doing you any good? Is your energy up? Is your weight down? Do you walk down the street with a spring in your step, a sparkle in your eye? If the answers to these questions are no, and you are ready to admit that the avalanche of diet books promoting an "eat more, weigh less" lifestyle (happy thought, but did it work?) are pie-in-the-sky and one-way tickets to diet disaster—then, ready, set, Energy Up! Whoo!

The Rules—and I'm Not Talking About Getting Married!

1. No Flour

Aha! Here it is. The first and possibly the most insidious and addictive powder of them all. Flour. Eat it up in pasta, in bread, in crackers. Feel it dull your senses, muddle your mind, make you sluggish. Watch it make you fat.

While people can usually see their way clear to giving up sugar and salt, they dig in their heels when it comes to giving up flour. You'd think it was un-American! Yes, I know: flour is in bread and bread crumbs, rolls, muffins, croissants, bagels, pancakes, waffles, and all the baked goods you can think of. (Come on, if you want to lose a few pounds, you shouldn't be eating these, anyway!)

Flour also is in pasta—at least the most common kind that we all grew up on, made from semolina wheat. I know all about pasta—it's the stereotypical Italian meal, right? And I should know . . . I always say, I'm half Italian—the bottom half! (Of course, I'm round on top now too, but I bought those!)

And I'm not just attacking *Italian* pasta either. When I say pasta, I'm including southern dumplings, Chinese wontons, Japanese gyoza and shumai, Jewish kreplach, Polish pierogi, and any other floury little balls of stuffed or fried dough. Like sugar and salt, white flour is one lethal little powder. If you've decided that you wanna put things in your body that are good for you, **GET RID OF IT.**

How did we get so hooked on flour, anyway? Let me show you the light.

Centuries ago, people used to grind their own grain into a highly nutritious coarse flour that was actually much better than what we're eating today (since no nutrients were removed, breads made from this flour didn't have to be "enriched" as they commonly are today). But it did spoil quickly and people began to look for a solution.

During the middle of the nineteenth century, they found one. Giant steamrollers had come into use which removed the wheat's "germ" (meaning the part of the grain with all the nutrients and healthy fiber); air sifters further "purified" it by removing the bran from the wheat, and white "refined" flour was born.

To the Victorians, this new, elegant white flour was considered far more desirable than the old, coarse brown stuff. Not only was it more stylish, but it didn't spoil as quickly as old-fashioned whole-wheat flour (a real consideration in the days before refrigeration!). And it caught on.

Today, adequate refrigeration is hardly the issue anymore, but white flour is still going strong. To counter the fact that white-flour breads are pretty much a nutritional wasteland, some companies have "enriched" the spongy, puffy, empty-calorie stuff with vitamins. Even so—it's still a stripped-down, overprocessed nightmare, totally devoid of fiber, that fills you up and leaves you panting for more.

And in case you're feeling the least bit virtuous—"Well, I only eat 'good' bread"—let me tell you that fine French bread is going to give you the same problems—and same cellulite—as Wonder bread. Neiman-Marcus's cookies are going to give you the same trouble as Chips Ahoy. Flour is flour, my friends!

There's another little "side effect" you also might want to think about: according to the experts (yes, I know, them again, but listen up anyway), lack of fiber (coupled with the huge amounts of white bread that most Americans eat) is thought to be a major contributor to the rise of colon cancer. Think about it! But what else could you expect from a white powdery substance?

Finally, wouldn't you like to see your energy level zoom **BIG-TIME?** Wouldn't it feel good to drop those thirty pounds you're lugging around, or is eating another sub or hero **THAT** important to you? You've tasted them before—now give my way a try.

I'm at the point where I am totally turned off when I see cake or bread or pasta—they're my enemies—and I know it! So why not accept that breads and pastas are off limits to you too, and see what happens? In the beginning, you may be horrified (many of my clients react the same way). But trust me here. **IT'S TIMES LIKE THIS THAT I REMIND MY CLIENTS THAT WE'RE PLAYING FOLLOW THE LEADER—AND I'M THE F@#!*ING LEADER! AND I KNOW WHAT I'M DOING.**

Breaking the bread habit is hard. Bread is considered such a basic—as pure as water—as good as bread, or so the old saying goes. Bread is synonymous with money . . . it's the staff of life . . . lovers crave a loaf of bread, a jug of wine, and thou . . . we ask God to give us this day our daily bread. Still, we don't live by bread alone, at least not on Planet Volta! Give it up!

Bread Between Your Lips? Next on Your Hips

When you go to a restaurant, what's the first thing they do? They put down bread—you reach for it. You probably have three pieces before you even get to your meal. It's quick, it's fast, it's the American way!—and it's a nightmare. It's probably **THE MAIN REASON** why women and men are walking around with extra weight. It's very difficult for me to get weight off people if they're eating bread . . . and hear me, girls, it's almost impossible to get rid of cellulite if you're not going to pass up the bread basket!

(Of course, if you're a young woman who has no problem with cellulite whatsoever, and aren't worried about ever getting cellulite in the future, forget about all this. Eat all the bread you want! But it'll catch up with you, sooner or later (it's not if, it's when!). Believe me, I work with women in their forties who were always naturally thin, never worked out a day in their lives, then suddenly their metabolism changed. All of a sudden, there are these lumps . . . cellulite . . . and they just don't know where to start. They usually say, "I've been eating like this since I was a kid, and it was never a problem." Well, guess what? Now it's a problem, **BIG-TIME!** Even if we're not quite sure why it happens, scientifically speaking—the reality is, it happens.

Pizza—Here's Pie on Your Thighs

Somewhere along the line, pizza got a reputation as a healthy food (the cheese gives you protein; tomatoes are a vegetable—so say the pizza makers!). But it's not. It's full of the things that drain your energy and add to your weight. The fact is, the advertising industry spends billions of dollars to brainwash people, to push their buttons (turn on your TV and really listen sometime!). I'm just saying, "Yo! You can't push mine anymore. I've been onto you for a long time!"

Strategies to Forget Flour

To be honest, I don't want you to strategize here. At least not until you're well along on your journey with me (and maybe never!). Don't write to me that you found rice-flour or corn-flour pasta in your local health food store, or spelt-flour bagelettes or flour-free muffins—and are those products "safe"? I'm not interested in the fact that soba noodles are made from buckwheat (*I know, I know*). *I just don't want to hear it.* Flour is flour, people! It's all white powdery stuff! (and even unbleached wheat or buckwheat flour is, at best, a sickly tan). **I WANT YOU TO LOSE THE TASTE, THE DESIRE, THE CRAVING, THE NEED TO STUFF YOUR FACE WITH BREAD AND PASTA.** I want to break the habit, kill the addiction, blow it out of existence and have you making different food choices!—not even thinking about foods made with flour, whatever kind of flour it may be!

Later—much later—you might want to **CAUTIOUSLY** experiment with products made from nonwheat flour, like rice-flour fettucine or corn-flour rigatoni. (Don't be fooled by so-called seven-grain breads, though. Usually they're mostly wheat, with barely a smidgen of the six other grains!) Let me tell you that for me, to this very day, all flour is off limits (remember, I want to kill the bread and pasta habit no matter what kind of flour it's made from). But if you must, see how *your* body reacts. If these products trigger your addictions and you start to bulk up, you've got your answer.

2. No Sugar

Let me be as in-your-face as possible here. Eating sugar (and I'm talking white sugar or brown!—same lethal stuff!) will not only cause you energy problems **BIG-TIME (DANGER! HIGH VOLTAGE!),** but is as addictive as all hell in the bargain. Eat sugar for quick energy, sweetie pie, and you're going nowhere fast. It lifts you up, brings you down—and leaves you with an insatiable craving for more.

One reason that sugar is such a problem is that our bodies were never meant to handle the 150 pounds or so that we're now consuming every year (that's over 30 pounds more than in 1975—according to figures assembled by the Department of Agriculture). Thousands of years ago, when we were a hunter-gatherer society, people ate foods that were "close to nature"—we had to! The foods our bodies were *meant to process* were vegetables, fruits, grains, and healthy fats (like those found in lean meats and nuts). But along with the advent of modern-day agriculture came processed sugar (as well as refined white flour and salt). **AND OUR BODIES SIMPLY CAN'T HANDLE THEM AND STAY HEALTHY!**

Sugar, people, is **NOT GOOD FUEL!** It has no nutritional value; in fact, it's a **TIME BOMB.** Over time, ingesting large quantities of sugar can lead to everything from obesity to adult-onset diabetes to heart disease! It ain't going to help you fly!

So what's the point? Why undermine your health and energy with this stuff? Why fill yourself up with junk that leaves you no room for healthy food **(GOOD FUEL!)** and is guaranteed to trigger strong, obsessive cravings for more? **WANT A LITTLE CHEMISTRY LESSON?** Hey, in a nutshell, for many people sugar triggers an eating binge: it starts off a chain reaction in your body which results in stored fat! In fact, the only other food that tells your body to store fat *is* fat. This means when you eat ice cream or sugar-frosted doughnuts or Oreos, or a gooey slice of coconut custard pie (which, once upon a time, used to send one of my clients to the moon and back!)—*you're eating a combination of sugar and fat which is sending your body a message with a double whammy!* Got my point? Good!

In my universe, when you reach for the **STAR,** no sugar means just that: **NO SUGAR!** No cakes, pies, or cookies. No ice cream, candy bars, sodas, and none of that weird "nonfood" like marshmallow fluff **(GET REAL!)**. Consider it gone. Ka-poof! It just doesn't exist anymore.

At the same time, you've got to be wary. Street-smart. I want you to be on guard against hidden sugars. **KNOW** where they are commonly lurking, ready to bring you down:

● In the jam or jelly you usually eat for breakfast. (No small loss: these days, there are terrific-tasting, all-fruit spreads right in the regular grocery store. Personally, I love them, and use them in many different ways—spread on a salt-free rice cake, spooned into plain, low-fat or fat-free yogurt, or drizzled on hot oatmeal, even, according to some of my clients, as a naturally sweet glaze on chicken or meats.)

● In ketchup. (Pour it on and you quickly pile up sugar—along with salt and calories. To be honest, I don't even like the word "ketchup" because of the ugly company it keeps—like greasy hamburgers and french fries! Let's delete it from our memory banks! Check out your local health food store for a no-sugar, no-salt variety, or better yet, substitute a salsa-style topping or a coulis [it's pronounced "coo-lee"]—a new word that I learned while researching this book: a coulis is a delicious seasoned puree from vegetables, fruit, or even meat or chicken juices.)

● Watch out for high sugar contents in fruit-filled yogurts (Dannon's Fruit on the Bottom regular yogurt has a whopping 44 grams of sugar, along with 240 calories and 140mg of sodium); in commercial salad dressings (tons of sugar!); in tomato sauces; and especially in breakfast cereals! And I'm not only talking about the obvious sugar-frosted, cocoa-puffed kid stuff either. There's even sugar (and salt!) in our supposedly safe grown-up favorites— like Rice Krispies, Corn Flakes, Cheerios, and good old Special K. Check them out . . . and cut them out!

Sugar, Sugar, What's What?
Granulated white sugar (table sugar) comes from crystallizing the juice of sugarcane or sugar beets, and is the most common form of sugar.

Dark brown sugar is simply table sugar coated with molasses for more "flavor" and color.

Crush *granulated sugar* (and add a little cornstarch) and you've got *confectioners' sugar,* which is also known as *powdered sugar.*

Corn syrup is liquid sugar made from cornstarch (it's got both glucose and fructose in it).

Molasses is the residue left after white sugar has been refined from raw sugarcane juice.

Sugar Strategies

I want to emphasize that I'm talking about *added sugar.* The white powdery stuff! Fruit, which also gives you nutrients and fiber, has *natural sugar* (called fructose), to satisfy your sweet tooth, and there's nothing wrong with that at all. Sweet little apricots, peaches, cherries, and plums and all the other fruits that God's good earth gives us are nature's own desserts and candies! I want you to cultivate your taste for these little jewels (see my list on page 106 for inspiration) and enjoy them at every meal. But if you go for frozen or canned fruit, watch out: be sure that no sugar has been added!

As for molasses, honey, maple syrup, corn syrup, and beet sugar, here's the scoop. They're bad news too: they provide calories and few vitamins and minerals, *and they have the same effect on the body that sugar does.* In fact, they're really just sugar in disguise. Raw, unrefined honey hasn't had all the nutrients processed out of it, so it has *some* value, but to be honest, if you have a sugar problem, it'll do the same things to you that sugar will.

What about Sweet'n Low, Equal, and other artificial sweeteners? Well, I can be reasonable, although in a perfect world, I wish you wouldn't use them either. But once you've gotten to the weight that you want and are maintaining it, if you have to, you have to (I have to admit, on occasion even I do). After a while, though, I predict you'll lose the taste for those chemical-filled, nasty little packets.

3. No Salt

The next point of my (soon-to-be-your!) guiding **STAR** is **NO SALT**—
and for many people, it's a threefold trap. First, processing adds salt—lots

of it!—to otherwise innocent foods. Next, we add even more during the cooking process at home. Finally, we douse food with salt **YET AGAIN,** at the dinner table! No wonder we're walking around puffy and bloated (and that high blood pressure and heart disease are on the rise!).

Now, I know that dealing with **NO SALT** may seem hard, but you can do it. (I did—and eventually, so do most of my clients. Cut salt from your diet and you'll start shrinking—immediately!)

Just don't delude yourself into thinking that salt is not **YOUR** problem. Even if you don't use salt when you cook, even if you wouldn't dream of touching the saltshaker at the table, don't imagine for a New York minute that you're eating a no-salt or even a low-salt diet. One woman I know, a glamorous cosmetics industry powerhouse, who **NEVER** cooked with salt—didn't even have it in her house!—insisted she already followed a fairly low-salt regime. Her eyes almost popped out of her head when I enlightened her about the "salt stalkers"—it's almost comical!—from 250mg in her morning cereal, 750mg in the soup she had for lunch, 900mg in the rice mix she served her family for dinner, 620mg in the Weight Watchers frozen dinners she threw in the oven on nights when she came home late from the office.

To stay healthy, our bodies do need some salt. Helloo—we can't function without it. It's what helps regulate the essential fluid content in our bodies (ever cut your finger and taste the blood? It's salty!). But salt (or sodium, as it's called on the food labels) occurs naturally in certain foods like celery, potatoes, and other vegetables, and in fish and shellfish. A hard-boiled egg gives you about 65mg salt, and you know that's natural! But I'm only concerned about the salt that's not natural, that gets *added* to foods.

This is where knowing how to read food labels comes into play. **Don't just check the nutrition facts—look for the list of actual ingredients on the package.** For example, an eight-ounce cup of Dannon nonfat plain yogurt, which **ONLY** gives you 110 calories, contains 150mg sodium (and 16 grams of sugar). But it's natural. If you look at the ingredients, there's no salt or sugar added—which is the key. Again, the sodium is natural (and the sugar listed is lactose, a natural component of milk). To help you keep up with what's in your foods, I highly recommend *The Supermarket Nutrition*

Counter, by Annette B. Natow, Ph.D., R.D., and JoAnn Heslin, M.A., R.D. It's a terrific paperback book that gives the calories, sodium, carbs, and fiber content of over eighteen thousand foods, from brand-name items to generic foods to your take-out favorites.

In addition, it's about a million-to-one shot that following my guiding Star you're going to reduce your intake of salt to anywhere near the point that it's detrimental to your health (if you're eating with Star Power, you'll certainly consume enough sodium naturally).

Give Us Some Numbers—How Much Is Too Much?

I think you'll be amazed at how little sodium the body actually needs in order to stay healthy, and how much you probably consume.

The fact is, the average American consumes 4000 to 5800mg of salt a day (about fifteen pounds a year), which is well over twice the recommended amount. In fact, even 2000 to 2500mg can be considered high, since in order to stay healthy, the same experts point out, our bodies only need about 500mg per day! Keep in mind, about one third of our salt intake occurs naturally in foods; the other two thirds (that we can easily cut out!) comes straight from either the processing or the shaker!

So where's the salt alert? Actually, everywhere! As with sugar, sometimes it's obvious—all over crackers, potato chips, popcorn, and other snacks. Pretzels can be low in fat but unless the bag says "no salt added," you're probably getting a hefty shot of salt with your munchies—maybe as much as 600mg in a single ounce (not to mention that they're made of flour—double whammy!). Salt is in most canned vegetables (and you can't wash it all off either), frozen foods (unless "no salt" is specified), and in fast foods **BIG-TIME!** I read recently that one fast-food chain's milk shake has more salt than an order of their fries! It's in your lunch: a bowl of Campbell's soup averages more than 800mg of sodium; a sandwich with a couple of slices of bologna, salami, ham, turkey, roast beef, or pastrami packs a wallop of about another 500mg (no matter how you slice it, this is salty stuff)! Care for some salt in your soda? You've got it—whether you want it or not. A single (twelve-ounce) can of Coke (diet or regular) gets you 50mg; in Pepsi, it's 35 mg. Guzzle a few of these every day and it adds up! And I can only assume that I *don't* have to warn you against baking soda and baking powder, since you're not going to be whipping up cakes and cookies anymore, are you? But yeah, they're damn salty too!

Be on the warpath against hidden salts. Here are some **DANGER! HIGH VOLTAGE!** salt traps:

- Luncheon meats and cured or smoked meats like hot dogs, bacon, sausage, ham, and salt pork. Also mousses and pâtés.

- Soups, especially the Asian ramen noodle soups. These innocent little meals are really salt mines in disguise (1000 to 1800mg in a single cup). Watch out for bouillon and clear broth soups. A cube of chicken bouillon has 1060mg of salt (whew!); a beef cube, 1120mg. I know—these numbers make a lot of eyes pop—not to mention sending blood pressures soaring! Bouillon packets aren't much better; they average about 860mg for either flavor.

- Pickled or marinated vegetables (unless they specify "no salt added," which, yes, I now actually find in my regular supermarket!—things are changing!). Capers, sauerkraut, prepared rice mixes, and almost all fast foods. I don't even have to mention shake-and-bake-type coatings for chicken or fish (over 500mg in two tablespoons), do I, because they're just seasoned **CRUMBS (FLOUR ALERT!),** guys!

- Cheeses (except the very few no-salt, no- or low-fat varieties—these have got to get better, people!). And if you're a cottage cheese eater, know that sometimes the low-fat version gives you less sodium than the no-fat version. When they take out the fat completely, they load it up with salt to make it taste "good." Besides, you can now buy low-fat, no-salt—which is what I use.

- Watch out for gravies, meat tenderizers, barbecue sauce, tartar sauce, and condiments like steak sauce (280mg sodium) or the spicy red cocktail sauce used with shrimp cocktails (two tablespoons give you 260mg!). In this company, Worcestershire sauce, at just 65mg of sodium a teaspoon (5 calories, no fat, and 1 lonely gram of sugar), sounds almost like a health food. Just don't pour it on!

• Finally, shun soy sauce like the salt plague. It packs 1000mg of sodium in a single, solitary teaspoon (and who uses one scant teaspoon?). It's simply liquid salt! Even the low-salt versions are a disaster—605mg is the sodium count on Kikkoman's "Lite" version. Teriyaki sauce? It's just soy sauce, people! Soy sauce with extra vinegar, salt, and sugar added! Absurd!

Truth in Advertising

Learn to read labels like it's a religion and you're born again—especially when it comes to scoping out sugar and salt. For example, I tell my clients to buy only products that have less than 100mg of added salt, although of course, this is not an exact science. As you get used to my program, use your newfound common sense. Tuna packed in water has 238mg (I'd like you to look for low-sodium kinds, which have about 40, but I'm not going to make you crazy over it). The 100-calorie fruit yogurt that I sometimes buy has 170mg of sodium. And plain, unflavored yogurt has 150mg—which is not added salt but natural, which actually takes it out of my realm of concern. We're only battling added salt, remember.

The fact is, salt is hard to avoid—I just want you to be wary and be aware. Ask for restaurant meals prepared salt-free (tell the waiter or waitress that you're allergic, and could actually pass out—it's the only way they'll take you seriously. Fear of a lawsuit works like a charm). Choose no-salt versions of your favorite foods whenever they're available, and avoid the obvious supersalty stuff, like chips, all processed foods, salty pickles, olives, and capers. Rule of thumb: If sugar or salt are among the first four ingredients on the package label, forget about it. If they're near the end of a long string of ingredients, chances are it's just a trace.

Shake the Salt Habit

If you think you'll miss salt, don't worry. As with sugar, it's a flavor that makes you crave more. The less you have of it, the more your palate will become used to the more subtle, natural flavor of foods. The *Chicago Tribune* (October 2, 1996) reported that researchers have shown that by limiting salt, you can actually lose the taste for it in two or three months—even to the point where you find it a turnoff.

For example, after just one week of High Voltage eating, one of my clients "cheated" with a chunk of fifty percent skim milk mozzarella cheese (370mg of sodium) and was amazed at how salty it tasted. Just remember, you really only need about one tenth of a teaspoon of salt per day, which is an amount you can accomplish all too easily since you get that much naturally in the foods you eat.

When you cut back on salt, you also open up a whole new world of creative cooking with spices, herbs, and other flavorings. Undercook your veggies and eat them crispy—they won't even need to be salted. Explore your spice cabinet and experiment with adding a little ginger and lemon to fish, or fresh basil to salads, tomato sauces, and omelets. Sprinkle a little cayenne pepper or onion powder on popcorn—but read the label carefully here. Don't take it for granted that your spices (like garlic pepper) don't have salt added. Often they do! *Read labels.*

I personally like food on the spicy side, so I'm delighted when our chef serves up dishes sparked with the assertive flavors of garlic, chives, curry powder, tarragon—and so are my clients. I've learned that a simple combo of finely chopped garlic, lemon juice, and coarsely ground pepper is a nice wake-up for many foods (try it over rice or grain). Or how about steamed couscous, topped with mushrooms, carrots, and other vegetables, with a touch of cayenne pepper, curry powder, freshly grated ginger, and a splash of lime juice? It doesn't have to be boring, baby! Use your imagination—but don't fall from your **STAR!**

Finally, if you *absolutely, positively* can't live another minute without the taste of salt (yecch!), there are salt substitutes on the market like Mrs. Dash, which is a salt-free seasoning; or Cardia, which, the company says, has fifty-four percent less sodium than table salt (sun-dried or Celtic salt, which is found in health food stores, is salt; it just contains the minerals that are extracted when common table salt is processed). Do I want you to go this route? **NO WAY**—although it may help you just to know that it is there. If you follow my **STAR,** though, we're going to be changing what you like, and salt will be a nonissue: hard to believe, but you won't want it—or like it—anymore. I sure don't!

Super Salt Substitutions

Because low-salt and no-salt diets have been used for years to help manage hypertension and high blood pressure, there are actually quite a lot of no-salt and low-salt products out there. Check them out (although if you're a heavy salt addict, not all of these products will taste too terrific at first). For example, now there are "no salt added" pickles and peppers (something I've never seen before!). I buy a no-salt hummus (regular hummus has 240mg of sodium) that I like to spread on rice cakes or eat with veggies—and it can't be beat. Just one tablespoon at a time, people. This is not until you've hit your happiest weight. Hummus can be like peanut butter for some people. Once they start, they can't stop.

4. No Processed Foods

All of my clients who recognized themselves as food addicts, others who have food-addictive tendencies, and even the one or two skeptics who practically choked on the word "addict" and can barely spit out "allergic" (but who nevertheless lost weight and kept it off following my **STAR**) have one thing in common. Processed foods and highly refined carbohydrates (which quickly convert to sugar) were once a big part of their diet. That's how the fourth point of my **STAR** came to be **NO PROCESSED FOODS.**

Now, we've already partly covered this in the previous three points, but **NO PROCESSED FOODS** takes it one step further. Chemicals, additives, preservatives, anything you might have difficulty spelling or pronouncing, **don't belong in your body.** I want you to eat as close to nature as you possibly can. Foods that come from the earth, the sky, and the sea. Fresh fruits and vegetables. Healthy organic chicken, turkey, and meats. Fresh fish and shellfish.

It means limiting foods that are frozen (they're usually off limits anyway because they're loaded with salt). It means steering clear of foods in boxes (think coffins), in plastic bags (think body bags), and in cans (think garbage cans). A good way to remember all this is to think: "Am I eating foods that are dead or alive?"

For example, is your breakfast a commercially prepared cold cereal?

That's **DEAD.** Is your lunch a frozen chicken pot pie and canned apple-cranberry sauce? It's **DEAD.** Or a hot dog on a bun, with sauerkraut, french fries, and a Coke? **DEAD AND BURIED, PEOPLE!** Do you snack on pretzels and cheesy crackers? **DEAD.** Are you opening up a box of pasta for dinner, to serve with canned tomato sauce, frozen broccoli, and cheese sauce? **DEAD, DEAD, DEAD,** and **DEAD.**

Run down the list below, and you may be surprised at just how many of your foods are **DEAD.**

Is Your Food Dead or Alive?
ARE YOUR VEGETABLES DEAD OR ALIVE?

1.	Raw vegetable salad with rice-wine vinegar dressing?	D	A
2.	Steamed asparagus with lemon and tarragon	D	A
3.	Frozen creamed spinach	D	A
4.	Canned baby peas and carrots	D	A
5.	Baked potato	D	A
6.	Grated red cabbage and carrots	D	A
7.	Frozen potato puffs	D	A
8.	Take-out coleslaw	D	A

Answers: DEATH TOLL: *Dead,* 3, 4, 7, 8. *Alive:* 1, 2, 5, 6. Frozen, processed, breaded, or doused in cream sauce, locked up and sealed in a can, or drenched in salt and mayo—all this kills poor veggies **BIG-TIME,** and may eventually kill you. Take your veggies straight: *in salad, steamed, freshly grated, or baked, with all the nutrients intact.*

ARE YOUR FRUITS DEAD OR ALIVE?

1.	Canned peaches in light syrup	D	A
2.	McIntosh apple	D	A
3.	Frozen blueberries	D	A
4.	Jar of applesauce	D	A
5.	Just-peeled banana	D	A

6. Slice of watermelon   D   A
7. Store-bought cherry pie   D   A
8. Mango puree splashed with lime juice   D   A

Answers: DEATH TOLL: *Dead,* 1, 3, 4, 7. *Alive,* 2, 5, 6, 8.
Once your taste buds get hooked on juicy, fresh fruit, tasteless canned, jarred, or frozen varieties with their overwhelming sugary syrups, additives, and preservatives will be the ultimate turnoff (why even bother with the calories?). And if you taste any real cherry flavor in a store-bought cherry pie—it's all syrupy sugary filling, starchy, high-fat crust—I'll eat that pie myself! (I'd probably pass out from the shock!)

ARE YOUR MEATS AND FISH DEAD OR ALIVE?

1. Organic beefsteak   D   A
2. Frozen Salisbury steak TV dinner   D   A
3. Sushi   D   A
4. Frozen breaded and fried fish fillets   D   A
5. Turkey roll   D   A
6. Smoked salmon   D   A
7. Frozen breakfast sausages   D   A
8. Fresh trout, broiled and splashed with lemon   D   A

Answers: DEATH TOLL: *Dead:* 2, 4, 5, 6, 7. *Alive:* 1, 3, 8.
Beware some "fatal" salt traps here, from frozen dinners and breaded or smoked fish to salty turkey roll and sausage. Stay alive with fresh beef, sushi (no salty pickled ginger, though!), and fresh trout.

ARE YOUR SNACKS DEAD OR ALIVE?

1. Glazed doughnut   D   A
2. Fat-free American cheese   D   A
3. Three Musketeers chocolate bar   D   A

4.	Bag of chips	D	A
5.	Slice of mushroom pizza	D	A
6.	Fresh strawberries	D	A
7.	Crackers-and-cheese snack pack	D	A
8.	Crudités with homemade salsa	D	A

Answers: DEATH TOLL: *Dead:* 1, 2, 3, 4, 5, 7. *Alive,* 6, 8.
Lots of coffins and body bags here—figuratively speaking, that is.
Watch out for cheese, even when it's fat-free (2, 5, 7), it's
processed and salted. And it's dough time with 1, 5, and 7 too.

If you haven't caught on to what I'm after here, I'm simply closing up a potential loophole. Hey, the U.S. Department of Agriculture might have been
wishy-washy about coming down hard on salt
intake (they did stick their necks out so far as to
suggest mere "moderation" with salt), most
likely because they were afraid of offending the
multigazillion-dollar processed food industry.
Hah! Not me! When you eliminate processed
foods, you automatically cut out a ton of hidden
salts and sugars. **And, people, you put yourself
back in command! Only by eliminating
processed foods are YOU in control of what
goes into your body!**

> **Volt-Note!**
>
> Processed foods fall so far afield of how people were meant to eat—yet have become such a staple of the American diet—that sometimes I feel that I must be in the Twilight Zone! *The Lifeline of America: The Development of the Food Industry* (see Bibliography, p. 270) points out that back in 1800, ninety-five percent of all Americans consumed minimally processed foods produced mostly on their own farms. But thanks to "progress," we just don't eat that way anymore! Our consumption of sugar and sweeteners has soared (sixty percent from 1909 to 1985); so has our consumption of fats. Instead of moving forward, people, we've developed a diet that's dragging us down—and doesn't work for us, at all. We are headed for a blackout!

5. Drink Water

**HEED MY CALL TO ARMS! WATER IS THE ULTI-
MATE WEIGHT LOSS WEAPON.** Get used to car-
rying little bottles of water around with you. For
some reason, drinking out of bottles is easier than out of glasses. Go figure.
No matter how you drink it, water is essential to my program. Six to
eight glasses daily (this is a good guideline for most people whether you want

to lose weight or not). At room temperature (easier to drink than icy cold!). I don't know exactly what it does or why, but damn, it works: you just lose faster when you're drinking it.

Some people say drinking water helps combat water retention. When you don't get enough, the body holds on to every drop. When you drink plenty of it, in effect you're sending your body a message: "Hey, let it go! There's plenty more where that came from." In addition, for some people it acts as an appetite suppressant, satisfying the desire to eat.

Water also has some **PRETTY TERRIFIC** cosmetic effects: it brightens your eyes, clears up your skin. Back in the days when Eileen Ford used to house fledgling models in her New York townhouse, she always said that she could tell who was drinking water and who wasn't by the clarity and texture of the girls' skin! That certainly made an impression on me.

On my program, you are going to be exercising **BIG-TIME.** Plenty of water keeps you from getting dehydrated. The American College of Sports Medicine advises water before, during, and after exercising to replace fluids lost through sweating. I agree. So drink!

Getting the Water Habit

Keep track of your water. Every time you finish a glass or bottle (I buy the eight-ounce sizes by the six-pack), make a little mark on a memo pad. If at the end of the day you don't see at least six, hopefully eight marks, you haven't done your job. Of course, in the beginning, drinking water is a lot easier for clients because I'm always there, nagging, reminding, shoving yet another bottle at them. But even when I'm not there, I want you to hear my voice motivating you!

Now, I'm not saying that drinking all this water is easy. But just make yourself **DO IT.** If you're not willing to give it a try, you're going to continue to be a very ordinary person . . . negative,

Volt-Note!

All this water isn't to be taken lightly either. The fact is, you're going to have to stay pretty near a bathroom wherever you go. It's one of the few downsides to my program—for me too! I try not to wear one-piece jumpsuits when I'm out shopping because they're so hard to get out of. But let me tell you—once you see it start working (one of my clients dropped three pounds overnight), once you start feeling better and more energy-driven, **YOU JUST DON'T CARE.** Like Nike says, "Just Do It!" Like High Voltage says, "Just F@#!*ing Do It!"

complaining, slightly unhappy with yourself and your life—slightly pudgy perhaps? And just basically all clogged up.

It all comes back to the same idea: If you're not ready for this, you're going to come up with a million excuses. If you've made the decision to do this, you're going to find ways to make it work. I'm giving you all the information you need, but you are the only one who can put it into action.

What's the Deal with Alcohol?

I really don't have much to tell you here. I can't drink. When I first start with them, my clients don't drink. If you can't go for one measly week without drinking, I say you have a different kind of problem (do you want to address that now or later?).

If you want to experience the full power of my program, **NO DRINKING** is a no-exception rule. Alcohol is full of sugars, which convert easily to body fat. The calories and sugar in alcohol count as much as the calories and sugar in food.

Now, I have had some clients who take a drink every now and then, and make no bones about it. Their weight has stabilized, they don't care to give up alcohol completely, but they do want their energy as high and vital as it possibly can be. Plus, they can have a drink without going for the whole bottle! Truth: I'm not happy about it because I feel they don't get the most Star Power benefits, but that's their personal choice.

If you can accept my **STAR** as your guide, following all the other points, and alcohol is a nonissue to you, then it's a nonissue. But let me just remind you about this: Alcohol *is* toxic; it congests the tissues, which makes the skin puffy (especially on your face, around the eyes). And in the long term, it makes your face sag. Even though we all know your friendly plastic surgeon can pull it back up for you, why accelerate the process?

Getting Off Alcohol

How to deal with it? Sweetie, unless you've got an alcohol problem (and if you do, I suggest you get yourself into a recovery program, pronto!), it's just not a big deal. You hardly need a fancy excuse these days to pass up the booze. People have tons of reasons for not drinking, from being pregnant to being health-conscious to simply not liking the taste. When I'm out to dinner and everyone is drinking wine or champagne, I have them put a bit of bubbly, sparkling water in my champagne glass. Some people say that drinking wine is just civilized. Well, maybe for you, but not for me. Not on my planet! If that's civilized behavior, you can keep it!

> **Volt-Note!**
>
> **S**ome people also say that a glass of wine (or any alcohol) may lower your risk of heart disease. Some other people say it also increases your risk of breast cancer! (not that I want to get into this endless verbal chess game). What I say: There are safer ways to fight heart disease—how about eating healthier and exercising?

Water and More

What else can you drink in addition to (not in place of!) your water? Milk—skim or the no-fat kind. After the first week of the program, try rice milk, soy milk, or almond milk and no-salt-added buttermilk (one of my favorites—and contrary to popular belief, it has no more calories than regular milk). If you like things rich and creamy—as I do—this can satisfy that taste. Fruit juice—although not too much. It has all the calories, but none of the fiber of whole fruit. Vegetable juice. Iced tea (no sugar please!). Herbal tea. Seltzer. Club soda (check to be sure it's salt-free). Coffee, iced or hot, if you want, or decaffeinated versions if you prefer. But I stay away from all sodas. Remember, even diet sodas have sodium in them. If you're drinking them by the six-pack, and are wondering why you're still puffy and bloated, that's why!

Now, turn your Star over and see **WHAT YOU CAN EAT.** The High Voltage lifestyle is about feeling happy, feeling energetic, and feeling satisfied—and eating the right foods makes all the difference.

6. Fruits and Vegetables

We've already talked about what you can't eat—and why (yecch! Who'd even want to eat that stuff?). Well, here's the good news. Fruits and veggies are things that you (almost) can't eat too much of! Have some fresh fruit salad at breakfast (keep a big bowl of it in the fridge). Grab a banana (loaded with potassium) or a bunch of red grapes for a snack. Serve up a rainbow platter of those good-for-you and delicious to boot orange, red, and yellow veggies that are creating such a beta-carotene buzz, like carrots, yams, and squash. And sweet potatoes, probably one of the most nutritious vegetables you can eat (besides being delicious). They're loaded with fiber, vitamins A, C, and more.

Think of fruits as nature's jewels. They have little or no fat, no sodium, not even a smidgen of cholesterol, loads of vitamins A and C, minerals, fiber—plus a naturally sweet taste. They've even got a high water content! You can't beat them for convenience (they don't need to be cooked), and accessibility (you can find an orange, an apple, or a banana at any corner grocery or deli—even 7-Eleven—whenever you need a fast snack). Plus, they're satisfying!

I've never had a client who found it hard to eat enough fruit. In fact, you almost have to be careful about eating too much! (I allow three fruits per day in the beginning; afterwards, don't go over four servings per day).

To me, any ripe fruit is "dessert." When I'm being supercareful—fanatic, actually—I usually go for the fruits that are lower in sugar, like strawberries, blueberries, Granny Smith apples, and pears, and leave sweeter fruits (like pineapple) for a special treat. If you buy canned fruits from time to time (or want to keep them in your pantry), be sure they're canned in water only (no syrup, not even "lite" syrup) and with no sugar added.

As for dried fruits—only when your weight is where you want it to be, and then *be careful.* Dried fruit can turn out to be a higher-calorie snack than you expect. For example, according to the University of California at Berkeley's *Wellness Encyclopedia of Food and Nutrition,* when fresh apricots are dried, not only is their natural vitamin C reduced, but their calories skyrocket! Three and a half ounces of dried apricots have 238 calories, while the same amount of fresh fruit has only 48 calories! Go figure.

Plus, if you've got a sugar thing, dried fruit can turn into a **BIG PROBLEM.** Those same dried apricots are more than forty percent sugar! Dried pineapple sometimes tastes like it's pure sugar! Dried fruits, delicious as they may be, can cause a sugar rush, crash, and craving that quickly turns into **WHO PULLED MY PLUG!** (That's certainly what it does to me.)

Fruits—Naturally Sweet

Apples • Apricots • Bananas • Blackberries • Blueberries • Boysenberries • Cantaloupe • Cherries • Clementines • Cranberries • Cranshaw Melon • Grapefruits • Grapes • Honeydew Melon • Kiwi • Lemons • Limes • Mangoes • Nectarines • Oranges • Papaya • Peaches • Pears • Persimmons • Pineapples • Plums • Pomegranates • Quince • Raspberries • Star Fruit • Strawberries • Tangerines • Watermelon

Bean Counting

They've got minerals, B vitamins, tons of fiber (remember, you're not eating bread!), protein (without any of the fat that you get in chicken and lean meat), and more. Plus, they're inexpensive, and tasty—what more could you ask? If you're eating beans as a side dish, half a cup is your serving size; as a main course (with veggies and a salad), go for a cup. Watch out for canned beans, though; they're usually packed with salt (most of which stays on even after rinsing).

Black Beans • Black-eyed Peas • Chickpeas • Kidney Beans • Lentils • Navy Beans • Red Beans • Soybeans • Wax Beans • White Beans (and more other beans than I could possibly think of)

Vegetables are even better for you than fruits. With more vitamins and minerals and plenty of fiber, low in sodium, crunchy, satisfying—they're winners all around. Red and yellow vegetables are important in our diet, but veggies like collard greens, broccoli, spinach, and kale are all high in vitamin C, calcium, iron, and more. The variety of vegetables is tremendous (and so are the ways to serve them!), so get brave: start venturing beyond the usual supermarket staples. Experiment with veggies you haven't tried before. (I love eggplant, for example, spiced and seasoned; it cooks up just like a steak!) Plus, experts have lots of kudos for vegetables these days (different types may help protect you against different diseases like heart disease, cancer, or stroke). I say go for them all! Three to five servings a day (plus three to four fruits) is what you're aiming for. Canned veggies? Never! Frozen? Only if they're frozen without salt—I know that many working moms depend on these because they can be cheaper than fresh veggies and keep longer, so if you have to, you have to. But I really want you to think about ways to get into buying fresh vegetables. How about saving money by buying your vegetables in bulk? If you live near a farmers' market, you can get some great prices on fresh vegetables that really beat the supermarket. One of my mother's friends makes a family outing of it: she and her children head to the local weekend farmers' market, pick out the freshest fruits and vegetables they can find, and when they get back home, they wash, cut, chop, cook, and put them in individual containers for the week ahead.

Vegetables—Your Mother Was Right

Artichokes • Asparagus • Bamboo Shoots • Beans (see list on p. 107) • Beets • Bok Choy • Broccoli • Broccoli Rabe • Broccoflower • Brussels Sprouts • Cabbage • Carrots • Cauliflower • Celery • Chilies • Collard Greens • Corn • Cucumber • Eggplant • Endive • Escarole • Garlic • Green Beans • Kale • Leeks • Lettuce (Arugula, Romaine, Boston, Bibb, Radicchio, Mesclun, etc.) • Mushrooms • Okra • Onions • Parsnips • Peas • Peppers (all colors) • Potatoes (all colors) • Rutabaga • Scallions • Snow Peas • Spaghetti Squash • Spinach • Sprouts (all kinds) • Squash • String Beans • Swiss Chard • Sweet Potatoes • Tomatoes • Turnips • Water Chestnuts • Watercress • Wax Beans • Yams • Zucchini

Sprouts

If you turned off sprouts years ago (when they were dumped on everything from salad to burgers to quiche), or if you've never tried them at all (even the word feels yecchy!), now is the time to give sprouts a second look. I go to the farmers' market and buy every kind of sprout I can find—mung, alfalfa—and put them in little plastic bags and munch them as a snack (they're like little bags of low-calorie, no-fat nuts!—really cool!).

How to Eat Five to Nine Servings of Fruits and Vegetables per Day

Eight A.M.

Either an orange, half a grapefruit, a slice of melon, strawberries, cut-up fruit salad, or a glass of freshly squeezed juice. That's serving 1.

One P.M.

Large mixed green leafy salad (that counts for 2 and 3), plus tuna or a hard-boiled egg. Plus a baked potato (that's serving 4).

Alternative Lunch:

Steamed or sautéed carrots, string beans, and broccoli over a grain like brown rice, couscous, or barley (the veggies count for 2 and 3). Plus a small green salad on the side (that's serving 4).

Six-thirty P.M.

Melon to start (5). Large mixed vegetable salad (that's serving 6 and 7). Grilled chicken breast and a vegetable (serving 8).

Ten P.M.

Snack: apple, strawberries, or other fruit (serving 9).

7. Poultry, Fish, and Lean Meat: The Protein Thing

I personally *love* the concept of being a vegetarian for spiritual reasons, and have tried it quite a few times. No luck! Inevitably I feel like my battery has gone dead. If you take in too little protein from other sources (easy if you don't have a full-time, ultracreative vegetarian chef), you may very well end up with an energy deficit.

Most of my clients enjoy fresh fish and shellfish—broiled, baked, blackened, grilled, steamed, just not drowned in butter, cheese, cream, or tartar sauce; chicken and turkey (white meat has less fat than dark—and skinless is always best!); and after the first week, even the occasional serving of lean beef or other meats.

I eat very little beef and lamb; however,

Volt-Note!

Fiber watch: This is as good a place as any for me to talk to you about fiber—which comes from plants, not animals. If you eat brown rice instead of white . . . oatmeal or a whole-grain cereal instead of Cocoa Puffs or Sugar Pops . . . a vegetarian meal or two a week (bean chili, for instance, instead of meat chili) . . . if you snack on fruit or popcorn instead of chips or cookies . . . you're adding fiber to your diet! As you might have guessed, High Voltage eating is naturally high in fiber (the National Cancer Institute recommends 25 to 35 grams of total fiber per day, to help reduce the risks of colon cancer and heart disease).

What does fiber actually do? One of its main effects on the body is that it helps prevent constipation—a problem that many of my clients have when they come to me. "No kidding," I always think, considering the way most of them eat! But I always ask them about regularity (it should be every day, people!), since most of the time they're all clogged up! To unclog, we start out with herbal teas—like senna tea, chamomile, flaxseed, comfrey, or goldenseal. What else helps: exercise; plenty of water; fresh fruits, veggies, and brown rice; and avoiding high-fat, salty dairy, white flour, and sugar (in short, the Star Power Plan!). Sometimes I'll recommend periodic colonics too—that's the Rolls-Royce of enemas, guys. Think of what Drano does to your sink—well, that's what a colonic does to your body!

if you still like the taste, there's nothing wrong with a burger now and then (just leave off the bun, please!) or lamb chop (trim the fat). Of course, once you're eating the High Voltage way, your lifestyle will be so healthy that the occasional serving of meat won't make that big a difference (and again, chances are you'll find a lot of it too rich and heavy, anyway).

I seldom eat pork roast or spareribs—too fatty for my taste—and I avoid goose and duck for the same reasons. I just don't like them. Sausage or bacon? Never—but those are a salt issue, anyway. The salt content in those foods—even when they're made with alternative ingredients like turkey—is comical. It may be turkey, folks, but it's salt up the gazoo! When I walk through an amusement park or street fair and smell the sizzling of greasy sausages and peppers, it actually nauseates me!

After the first week, if *on occasion* you want to add meat to your diet, I see no problem with that. (Every once in a while even my body—lily-pure as it is these days—seems to call out for calves' liver. I guess it thinks I need the iron!) But "on occasion" means just that, people—not every day or even every week.

About veal: I totally lost my appetite for veal when I learned of the horrendous and inhumane way veal calves are raised! They are penned up in a teeny, tiny space, unable to move, and fed nothing but milk (veal needs to be snow-white and any movement on their part could build muscle, which might make a pink streak in the veal). It's almost a blessing that they are put out of their misery and their hellish lives in such a short time.

The main thing I want to tell you about in this section is portion size. **WATCH IT!** Our eyes have become accustomed to servings that are double, sometimes even triple what we should be eating. A good rule of thumb I learned recently: A three-ounce portion should be the size of a deck of cards or the palm of your hand. A serving of chicken on the bone is a quarter of a chicken—not a half or a whole bird! (Poultry and meat give us pro-

they somehow seem to disappear in one fell swoop (at least that's the case in *my* house). How to use them: Once your weight is where you want it to be, add a few blanched almonds to a salad for extra crunch, or some chopped walnuts on top of plain yogurt and strawberries, or use one-ounce packs as on-the-go snacks.

9. Dairy Products

For a while, I tried taking all the dairy out of my diet because I was concerned about all the hormones they give cows these days. That's the reason I try to introduce my clients to some alternative milk products, like soy milk or rice milk. Rice milk, in fact, which is sweeter than regular milk (use it in your coffee and you'll never ever miss sugar!), is actually one of my favorite treats; I can't recommend it highly enough. You can find it these days not only in health food stores but even on your regular grocer's shelf.

But milk is not one of those things I'm going to battle over. My clients enjoy skim milk, no-salt or low-sodium cheeses (when they can find them), low-fat, salt-free cottage cheese, and nonfat yogurt. These are some of the most efficient ways for women to take in calcium, which you need to build bones and to help prevent osteoporosis.

Even so, as healthy as your diet may be, the fact is, if you're not a big milk drinker and if you don't eat much yogurt, it's still going to be hard to get all the calcium you need. Even if you're eating other calcium-rich foods (like spinach, sardines, and oranges), milk does it best. It's now recommended that women over twenty-five get at least 1200mg of calcium per day, so I strongly recommend talking to your doctor or nutritionist if you think

---

Volt-Note!

What about peanut butter and other natural nut butters (like cashew butter, almond butter, pecan butter)? Not for the first week. Not when weight is still an issue. But definitely within the possibility of a High Voltage lifestyle once you've reached your goal (do I hear a sigh of relief out there?).

So here's how to test the waters: Buy a jar of unsalted, no-sugar peanut butter (or whatever nut butter is your favorite), and allow yourself a tablespoon on a rice cake (no more than once a day, please!). If your weight doesn't go up after a week, if you aren't tempted to devour the whole jar at a single sitting, you're probably on safe territory.

But be forewarned: Even I can't keep these around. Somehow, the whole jar just disappears. And when you live alone, like I do, there's no one else to blame! And it's too bad, because the last time I bought a jar of peanut butter, a day later it was gone. I got frantic because I figured someone had broken into my apartment and eaten it all. Some thief! Left the TV. Left the VCR. Ate the peanut butter. Left the spoon. Reality check!

you're going to need an appropriate supplement! To be absolutely honest with you, I started taking calcium supplements—and recommending them to my clients—after doing the research for this book.

10. Grains for Your Brain

When people cut out pasta, I flatter myself that after a few weeks they barely miss it because they've opened their eyes to the world of fresh, delicious grains—low in fat, cholesterol-free, with plenty of fiber and all the appropriate minerals and vitamins. Fortunately, the taste (and health value!) of grains have caught on so much in the last few years that a lot of you are already eating brown rice and basmati rice, as well as discovering couscous, quinoa (pronounced "keen-wa"), barley, and other goodies.

Be careful with grains. We're talking starch here, and once a day is enough while you are trying to lose weight. The grain issue also reminds me again about how we've lost our sense of reason in regard to portion size. A side order serving of grain is half a cup, cooked—not dry. That's it! If the grain is your main course player—go for a cup.

Grains cook up for breakfast, can be tossed in a salad, seasoned and spiced for a side dish or main dish too (just like pasta, people, except this stuff is good for you and doesn't seem to be as addictive). Some top grains? Brown rice (old faithful—you can get it anywhere, even in many Chinese restaurants). Wild rice. Aromatic rice like basmati—a staple of Indian diets (whole-grain basmati rice is not processed!). There's buckwheat groats (when these are roasted before boiling they're known as kasha). Bulgur is a Middle Eastern grain—wheat kernels are steamed, dried, and cracked into small pieces (it's the grain you find in tabouli!). Pass up the white, pearled barley that you find in most supermarkets. It's been refined—**THAT MEANS PROCESSED.** Instead, there's brown, unpearled whole-grain barley (you can find it in most health food stores).

As we look beyond pasta, new grains are turning up all the time. Lots of unusual, ancient grains, like spelt and kamut, are being brought to us by small companies around the world. **TRY THEM—YOU MIGHT LIKE 'EM** (hey, until recently, like most people, I had never even heard of these—but now that I have, I'm excited!). So be adventurous! Explore! And while you're doing this, remember that you're also creating a demand which just might make big business sit up and take notice and give us more nutritionally valuable foods and less **GARBAGE.**

TRUST ME—when you create a demand, big business responds. Look, I really don't think people sit around purposefully trying to poison our bodies, but the fact is, it's profitable! So let's demonstrate a new way to be profitable—one that's safe, healthy, and gives them the same bottom line! As I always say, welcome to the **VOLT**-Age!

> **⚡ Volt-Note! ⚡**
>
> I don't think for a minute that big companies are in cahoots, thinking up ways to strip our foods and rob us of nutrients. In fact, many times, they do try—and we let them (and ourselves!) down. In all fairness to McDonald's, they do offer salads; they did come out with a healthier burger, the short-lived McLean, which the public rejected. So take a stand, create a demand, join the cosmic command! Energy Up! Whoo!

Build Your Brain, Eat Lots of Grains!

Amaranth • Barley • Basmati Rice • Brown Rice • Buckwheat Groats • Bulgur • Couscous • Kamut • Kasha • Millet • Oats • Spelt • Triticale • Wheatberries • Wild Rice

Taking Vitamins

If I ruled the planet, there would be no processed foods and everyone would be eating fresh fruits and vegetables, whole grains, organic meats and poultry, very little fat, and drinking water by the gallon—and getting our vitamins and minerals from the food we eat. Energy up! Whoo!

Reality check: that ain't gonna happen. In the real world, it's almost impossible to get enough vitamins and nutrients with the highly processed, chemically saturated, nutritionally altered food we eat (dead food)—not to mention the convenience food–oriented lives that many of us lead.

Even if you're following the Star, the fact is, your daily calorie count would soar outta sight if you tried to get the recommended daily requirements from food alone. According to the *Nutrition Action Newsletter,* in order to get enough calcium, for example, you'd have to drink three cups of milk . . . or eat six cups of yogurt . . . or four pounds of spinach . . . or eighteen oranges . . . or thirty-six cans of sardines, **EVERY DAY.** Hellooo! I don't think so! (For those of you who don't know it, this terrific newsletter is put out by the Washington, D.C.–based Center for Science in the Public Interest, the nonprofit consumer watchdog group that blew the whistle on movie theater popcorn, fat-free muffins, Chinese food, and a ton of other things. Three cheers—and a whoo! for them!)

A hundred and fifty years ago, a higher daily calorie count was possible—without ballooning—because people weren't as sedentary. In fact, they actually consumed far more calories (and fats) than we do now, but managed to stay a whole lot leaner (not hard when you wake with the sun and put in a long hard day on the family farm).

But society changed—we got hooked on sugars and processed foods and fats, became a whole lot less active as we moved from the farms to cities and towns—and we just can't take in all those calories anymore.

But we still need the nutrients. That's why, practically speaking, it's a good idea to talk to a nutritionist or your doctor about vitamins and a nutritional supplement. While nothing replaces Mother Nature, this is just common sense! Bingo! When I have my vitamins and supplements on the market (hey, I'm working on it), I'll be sure and let you know.

High Voltage's **Ten Commandments**

(Until my program is second nature to you, copy this page, tuck it in your wallet or purse, and keep it as a reminder.)

1. **NO FLOUR:** Avoid anything made with flour, especially wheat flour (like breads and bread crumbs, crackers, baked goods, and pastas).

2. **NO SUGAR:** Stay away from sugary treats like candy, cookies, cakes, and other junk foods. Watch out for added sugars in salad dressings, tomato sauces, and breakfast cereals!

3. **NO SALT:** Steer clear of salty snacks. Watch out for hidden salts in soups, cheese, packaged rice mixes, soy sauce, and other condiments.

4. **AVOID PROCESSED FOODS:** Eat as close to nature as possible! Stay away from foods that come dumped in a box, crammed in a can, stuffed in a bag, or wrapped in plastic—they're loaded with chemicals and additives and addictive sugars and salts.

5. **DRINK WATER:** Without water, there is no life. Without water, *this plan will not work.* Make it at least six to eight full glasses a day, more if you can!

6. **FRUITS AND VEGETABLES:** Open season here. Enjoy all of nature's best— at least five to nine servings daily.

7. **POULTRY, FISH,** and **MEAT:** Eat skinless chicken and turkey, fish, shellfish, and occasionally lean cuts of meat. Steer clear of sausage, bacon and all processed luncheon meats, fatty marbled beef, goose and duck. Another protein source: eggs (but no more than two a week if you're watching cholesterol).

8. **FATS:** A tablespoon of olive oil or other vegetable oil per day is fine. Beware of fats that are solid or semisolid at room temperature. Butter, margarine, lard, and shortening are all no-no's.

9. **DAIRY PRODUCTS:** Stick with no-fat milk, skim milk, no-salt-added buttermilk, low-fat (no salt) cheeses, and nonfat yogurt, please.

10. **GRAINS:** In moderate portions (½ cup servings) eat brown rice, wild rice, millet, couscous, barley, kasha, and other whole grains.

ENERGY UP! WHOO!

Chapter 6

POWER SURGE!
THE HIGH
VOLTAGE
WORKOUT

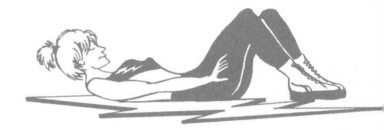

"Exercise? *I want to but I don't have the time to fit it in. There aren't enough hours in the day."*

How many times have you said this—and how many times have I heard it! (Don't ask!) Well, sweetie pie, we're going to *find* the time for you! Let me tell you—and I know you've heard it umpteen times in your life, but maybe I'm the cosmic commander that can convince you **HOW IMPORTANT, HOW NECESSARY, HOW VITAL WORKING OUT IS FOR A HEALTHY, HIGH-ENERGY, HIGH-PERFORMANCE LIFE.**

You gotta do it. You gotta take the plunge. There are twenty-four hours in the day—and I'm asking you to devote just one of them (not necessarily all at once either!) to exercise. To walking around the block or on a treadmill. To running. Or swimming. Or jumping rope. Or biking. To signing up for an aerobics class or working out to an at-home video. *To whatever turns you on.* You say nothing turns you on? Well, I don't believe it; you just haven't found what turns you on yet. It's *my* job to help you find it.

You don't need to join a gym or buy expensive equipment either. All you've gotta do is get moving. You don't have to wait till you lose weight. Any *body* can put one foot in front of the other and get into walking (which happens to be the best and most accessible type of exercise there is). In fact, the biggest weight loss I was ever part of was with a New York client, a high-powered public relations guy who was about a hundred pounds overweight. All we could do together, *literally,* were the most basic stretches in the morning and a slow half-hour walk at the end of the day. But we did it. And he got into it! (P.S. He went on to lose the hundred pounds, worked up to an hour-and-a-half walk, got into karate—see, we found what turned him on!—and he's now a dedicated black belt!)

What's exercise gonna do for you? (I hear this a lot too: all that "What's in it for me?" bullshit). Well, what's *not* in it for you? *It's all for you!* With exercise, you get the most bang for your buck. You'll feel more alert. More energetic. Stronger, fitter, and less tired. You're gonna look better—before you even lose so much as a pound, you're gonna look *thinner* (that's because toned muscles look leaner and more streamlined, people, than flabby ones!).

Think of it this way: On one side of the scale you've got a toned, in-shape body, more energy, higher self-esteem, stress relief, weight loss, plus pretty solid preventives against heart disease, osteoporosis, and even possibly breast cancer. Experts say you'll even sleep better! On the other side—overweight, fatigue, flabby muscles, sluggishness . . . I say, *no contest!* Do you need to wait for that first heart attack in order to get with it? I tell my clients to pretend they've had that heart attack already—and are now going to start living their lives at their fullest, and healthiest!

Finally, there's something about an aerobic workout—to music that turns you on—that has a lot to do with the transformational part of my program. Remember, working out with music played a gigantic role in my transformation!—and it can in yours too.

Music—the Heartbeat of My Workout

I've always said that if you want to stay mentally and physically young, follow the music scene of the day (this is no small issue!). And if you want to get turned on to fitness in a whole new way—and stay turned on—music can be a powerful motivating factor. Music is the heartbeat of all this because you've got to love working out—or you won't keep it up. Whether they realize it or not, ninety-nine percent of the people who are attracted to me are music-driven; they just wouldn't work out as hard, as fast, without the music blaring.

> ### Volt-Note!
> ### High Voltage's Workout
> ### Music Suggestions
>
> - Volumes 2, 3, and 4 of *Dance Mix USA*
> - RuPaul's *Foxy Lady*
> - Tape your local radio station's dance music mix
>
> Play any of the above as loud as possible when you work out.

One of my Boston-based clients even gave a name to the high he gets from working out to music: he calls it the "eye of the tiger," after the song from one of the *Rocky* movies. When I speak to him to check in on his energy level, I always ask if he got the eye of the tiger that day. That heart-thumping, transformational, almost hypnotized feeling is what keeps him hooked on working out. (If you have an addictive personality, then all you can do is to change what you're addicted to.) But know this: *the feeling you get from working out to music is addictive!*

> ### Volt-Note!
>
> Peter Gabriel, the huge pop star, not surprisingly immediately understood the power of working out to music. His agent and mine, ICM's Jonny Podell, gave Peter a workout session with me when he was in New York, and he really clicked into my Energy Up! Whoo! As for me, I was astounded by how strong Peter was aerobically. Of course, he would be, because when he does one of his concerts, he's jumping all over the stage! When Peter went to one of his homes in Europe (and he has quite a few!), his secretary called Jonny wanting to know what all this High Voltage "Energy Up! Whoo!" was about. Good for him, I say! He just didn't stop whooing! He's a true cosmic commander!

If you can't get into contemporary music, then look to whatever turns you on—country, jazz, fifties rock 'n' roll, Motown, big-band music, disco. I find that people are usually turned on to the music of their youth (High Voltage appeals to the kid in all of us), or whenever they were feeling their fittest and most attractive. Even if you think I'm crazy (actually, I am), I want you to go to your local music store so you can really remember what used to get you moving—because, I repeat, music has a gigantic role in recharging your life.

One of my favorite clients, Denise Rich, a stunning and sexy brunette with a trim, curvaceous figure, also really gets it (of course, she *is* a supersuccessful songwriter!). In fact, one of the most inspiring spots in the world for working out is in her magnificent penthouse overlooking Central Park, which has the most incredible sound system! When we work out together, we keep the decibel level so high that her household staff boogies to the beat as we literally rock the whole apartment. Of course, that apartment is two full floors of the building (and no one's complained, yet!). The energy has even spread to her doormen—when I walk in, they all yell, "Energy Up! Whoo!"

Denise finds music a terrific release. She says it helps her deal with the enormous pressures of her daily life, which includes writing songs for hit films, being part owner of a recording company, doing tons of charitable work—and being a terrific mom!

The energy release you get from aerobics and, specifically, my Power Surge Workout (more on that later) and my "Whoo!" are part of the reason that I'm not that fond of the health club scene. The Whoos my clients and I release are so powerful that they can be disruptive to other exercisers **BIG-TIME.** Some people, especially if they're shy or reserved, might even find the exuberance of the High Voltage workout and Whoo! a bit odd or embarrassing, even in the privacy of their own homes. If that sounds like you— *you've still gotta do it!* You've gotta release that energy. Part of the reason I'm so calm and sleep like a baby most nights is because I get rid of any pent-up negative energy during the day.

When you start getting out your negative energy and strengthening your aerobic ability, the high you get is more powerful than any drug on this planet (and believe me, I've tried them all!). That's what the high in High Voltage is all about! Plus, as I always say, High Voltage is not just what the program is called. I *am* High Voltage—and I want to transmit it to you! So plug in!

Believe It or Not: I Hate to Exercise

Before we go any further, there is something I should make clear: I hate working out! I think I created my whole business—my whole lifestyle—for two reasons: number one, in order to listen to dance music all day, and number two, so I would have people to work out with. Otherwise, I'd just have to hire me—and I can't afford me!

My clients are often amazed that when we work out, I do everything they do—from the Power Surge Workout to the bike rides, beach walks, and then some (massages and facials included—poor baby, it's a tough life!). Some trainers may stand there and tell them what to do. But I'm an energy conductor: I actually *do* what the clients do! It's one of the reasons that I like to make sure I have different clients who like doing different things. It keeps it fun for me—and "fun" is a very important word in my vocabulary.

Sometimes, my working out alongside a client actually embarrasses them, especially some of my clients in their twenties who are huffing and puffing while I'm still going strong—don't forget, I'm fifty. I'm working with a beautiful twenty-something singer now and pushing her past her bounds—and she's loving it. Model Beverly Peele told one broadcast journalist, "It's ridiculous. [Voltage is] twice my age and I can't keep up with her." My favorite answer to anyone having difficulty working out with me is to tell them to keep at it: If you do, when you get older you can be as fierce and fabulous as I am.

Power Surge: It's Tough, but It's Easy (I'll Explain)

To make my program work, you need to commit to a daily aerobic activity—at least thirty minutes—and whenever you need a recharge of high-powered energy, do a High Voltage Power Surge Workout. I'd love it if you could do Power Surge every day; I've done it every day for years. Before I began my Spa Weeks, I sometimes did it **ALL DAY**—there were times when I worked out with up to seven people in a single day! How did I hold up? Well, as they say, energy promotes energy! Energy is a muscle. If you don't use it, you lose it!

The more you do, the more you can do—that's one of my mantras. And I've done my workout everywhere. One of the most fabulous places I ever did it was on the top deck of a yacht! We were on the StairMaster when the yacht hit rough waters—it was a most unusual feeling! And really cool!

Along with eliminating the three deadly white powders from my diet (the base of the Star Power Plan), I credit Power Surge for the shape—and health—I have today.

Power Surge and Star Power—they go hand in hand. You may lose weight on Star Power, but you won't feel the real High Voltage energy rush unless you get your body moving. Everyone from the gym teacher at your local Y to the experts at the Center for Eating and Weight Disorders at Yale University agrees that physical activity is essential to successful *maintained* weight loss.

What that means: While exercising won't make that much difference in your initial weight loss, *it's what helps to keep the weight from coming back* by stepping up the pace of your metabolism. Exercise is what helps my clients' bodies adjust to needing less fuel (i.e., food). If your body wants to weigh more, exercise is what kicks your metabolism into a higher gear.

Power Surge is intense. But I developed it in order to give my clients the best—and fastest—results (you want slow results, go elsewhere!). When you charge the kind of money I do, you gotta get results fast, thank you very much!

There's nothing fancy or complicated about the exercises in Power Surge. In fact, I'm betting in part on the familiarity factor in order to get you to try this and make it part of your life (I'm sure you're going to recognize quite a few of the moves). The fact is, while it's a damn tough workout (most beginners and nonexercisers barely get through the warm-up!), it's also easy (I'll explain, I'll explain).

Power Surge is accessible . . . and I like it that way. *Any body* can do it, anywhere . . . it adjusts to your own body, your own needs, and your own pace. That's because I don't believe in tricky choreography or fancy moves that only a professional dancer could do. Surprised? Well, even though I'm coordinated, I just don't like that stuff. I'm not here to intimidate, I'm here to motivate!

Plus, Power Surge is broken down into sections for you—ten minutes of stretches, twenty minutes of floor work, ten minutes of arm exercises, and twenty minutes of kick-ass aerobics. (Power Surge has twenty minutes of aerobics because it's part of a one-hour program. I really want you to do thirty minutes of aerobics every day whether or not you do Power Surge.) This makes it easy to incorporate the exercise elements you want, and need, into your daily life and schedule. One client of mine, for instance, fits in her daily half hour of aerobics on her home treadmill (I *insist* on making that aerobic half hour part of your life!), and she does ten minutes of Power Surge stretches every day to keep limber and flexible. Another client walks every morning—and does my Power Surge upper-body workout three times a week (his arms are in great shape!). Whenever clients need a real energy boost—and want to drop a few pounds fast—they do the full Power Surge Workout every day for a week! The results show too!

My goal is just to get you moving and to get you to make working out a nonnegotiable part of your new life.

In fact, some people may even find my workout a bit old-fashioned (I do get a chuckle out of that). Well, maybe it is. There are no gimmicks here; this is not the latest fad. These are the same classic moves I've been doing for years. **They worked then, they work now.**

The roots of my workout go way back! In fact, the second time I made the cover of the *New York Daily News* was in 1986, the year the Mets won the pennant and I was working out with the players' wives at the Excelsior, then one of the most exclusive—and expensive—private health clubs in New York. This was during my high glitter period. (Of course, after a while, the glitter act did wear a bit thin—even though I didn't realize it at first. It was only after Andy Warhol told me that my message may not be getting through that I began to tone it down. "People may have a hard time getting past what you look like," he told me. Although I had heard that many times before, *him* I listened to. I figured he knew what he was talking about. If I looked extreme to him, I can only imagine the effect it had on others.)

Working out with the Mets' wives, I met Dani Mazzilli, baseball player Lee Mazzilli's wife (Lee is known as one of the cutest guys in baseball!). She and I became best buddies for a time and did regular six-thirty A.M. workouts together in her little office at Fox, where she worked as one of the hosts of *PM Magazine*. That's where I met Matt Lauer, now of course the gorgeous co-anchor of the *Today* show, but then showing up for his very first day on the job as Dani's co-host. Matt walked in on us in the middle of a workout, both spread-eagled on the floor, and to tell you the truth, he looked a bit stunned (to be fair, this was the height of my glitter era— lightning bolt makeup, sequin leg warmers, hot-pink and turquoise leotards, and feathers in my hair). "Welcome to New York," Dani and I both chirped! Energy Up! Whoo!" P.S. Matt's a great guy! Thank God he had a sense of humor.

One Hour, Total Fitness

Of course, if you've got the daily hour to devote to fitness (and quite a few of my clients do), I'd like to see it become part of your daily life. In one single hour you get it all: a basic stretch to warm up muscles; aerobics to get your heart pumping and your blood flowing; upper body strengthening, abdominal work, and basic floor work (which means legs, hips, and butt).

And that's just the warm-up! After the first hour, then we really get to work! (No, I'm not kidding—I just aim high!) Perfect world: I'd like you to do Power Surge, then twenty minutes to an hour of pure aerobics—walking, running, treadmill, StairMaster, whatever you choose.

Reality check: Do what you can . . . even if it's just fifteen minutes a day. Some is better than none. Tip: Add more of what inspires you: more weight training if that's your high, more crunches if you really want to get those abdominals in shape, more aerobics if you want to lose weight. And always, louder, faster music to help you soar—rock, jazz, country, show tunes, a Sousa march, whatever turns you on. If your roommates, family, or neighbors complain, get headphones! I said it before—music is the heartbeat of all this! You've got to love doing it—or you won't keep it up.

(Me, I like the heart-pounding beat of the old disco classics or current dance music—remember, I come from the nightclub world, not the health club world. I can't wake up without that beat—I turn my radio on, even before breakfast. And anytime I start feeling my energy drop, the music goes on and it's Energy Up, Whoo! Whoo!)

Any Body **Can Do It!**

As I said, Power Surge is tough—not because the moves are hard, but because it's thorough and it *works your whole body*. That's why *any body* can do

energy up!

it, at any level. Sometimes, when I'm working out with a new client, they look up from their crunches and say, "I don't believe I'm paying you for this!" But I know my clients wouldn't be working as hard if I wasn't there alongside them, urging them on. No way! It's moments like that when I like to joke that they're not my clients, they're my victims!

Volt-Note!

It was during my glitter period that the Excelsior Club became my home base. I even did a segment there for Robin Leach's *Lifestyles of the Rich and Famous* show (yes, I even got him to whoo!—kind of). At the time, I attached many of my energy concerts to charity functions such as Easter Seals and MS, and it was during one of these events, at the Excelsior, that I met fitness guru Richard Simmons. He was doing publicity for his workout tape *Gray Foxes*, which featured celebrity parents like Farrah Fawcett's mother, Al Pacino's mother, and Sly Stallone's mom, Jackie. Well, the women were so enthralled with my clip-on glitter hair pieces covered with multicolored sparkles that I took the clips out of my hair and put them in theirs. Jackie Stallone and I are friends to this day. In fact, when Jackie and I see each other, we both yell Whoo!

As for Richard, he didn't quite know what to make of me then. But he was from California, and this was my town, New York! I've watched his career for years and admired him because, like me, he lives it and believes it and truly wants to spread the word. We've both got our hearts in the right place! You go, Richard!

But it's all in fun. There's actually a very powerful tête-à-tête that goes back and forth when a client turns the reins over to me. As I said, everything in our relationship is predicated on the fact that we're gonna play follow the leader—and you know who that is!

You Can Do More than You Think

One of the first things I do before a workout with new clients is assess their fitness level. I do this with a number of basic exercises: push-ups to test upper-body strength, jumping jacks for aerobic ability, plus a standard touch-your-toes stretch to see their flexibility level. These tests are individual and have nothing to do with weight. In terms of flexibility, for example, some of my trimmest clients are models who are as stiff as a board; I also had a client who was seventy pounds overweight and as flexible as Gumby!

I divide my clients into three different categories of flexibility: 100-watt (high), 60-watt (average), or switched-off (low). If you want to see where you are, stand with your feet slightly apart and your knees only slightly bent (not locked), lean over, and touch your toes. A high-wattage score means you can touch your toes with ease. Maybe you can even put

126

your palms flat on the floor. You're very flexible. If you're 60-watt, you can probably get within a few inches of touching your toes. That's about average, in my experience. Switched off? You can't get much past your knees, if that. But don't beat yourself up about it. You can only improve.

If you want to test your upper-body strength, as I do with my clients, do the same thing with push-ups (unless there is a medical reason not to, I have clients do them men's style, no bent knees allowed). And I choose push-ups because everyone has a basic idea of how to do them.

I admit that push-ups *are* hard, especially for women, who usually need to work on their upper-body strength. How do you rate? I find most women can barely do one—that's switched off. If you can do up to five, give yourself 60 watts—a good-to-average score, as far as I am concerned. From six to twelve push-ups is *very* good—that's a 100-watt score. Congratulations! Something to strive for? Twenty-five push-ups. In my book, that's a real high-energy score! Note: If you can't manage even one men's push-up, don't be discouraged. Try women's push-ups, with bent knees, with the same scoring ratio, and see how you do.

Next, I put the music on and ask my clients to get on a treadmill, StairMaster, or any other piece of aerobic equipment. This gives me a sense of their energy level so I can determine how fast or slow our workout music should be. If the beat is too fast, they'll knock themselves out; if it's too slow, they won't be pushing hard enough. If you want to try this at home, march in place, run up and down a flight of stairs, or try jumping rope. Just be sure you don't choose music that is too fast—you'll simply knock yourself out before you start. This is something you'll have to play with.

With clients, of course, I'm putting them through a pace that they never thought was possible—it's like boot camp. Readers at home: I want you to check with your doctor first before starting, and don't get stuck on assessing your level by yourself. You'll only get stuck. The key thing is to get started, no matter what level you're at. (One of the hardest things about bringing my workout program to you is to get you to start—it's understanding the motivation factor. That's why I'm beating you over the head to work out to music, especially if you're a true beginner who hasn't exercised in years. You need it—even if you only use it to dance around your apartment in the beginning!)

Trust me, you're not going to stay with Power Surge—or any other workout program—unless you do it to music. **AS I SAID BEFORE, I'M NOT PSYCHIC BUT I KNOW WHAT I'M TALKING ABOUT HERE!**

I've observed that many women seem to need the "push" that trainers give them, more so than most guys. Many but not all women seem to have more of a preconceived notion as to their physical limitations, especially if they're older—often they underestimate what they can do. This is not always an age thing either; I've seen nineteen- and twenty-year-olds who are not used to pushing themselves. Men who once played team sports when they were kids, with a coach busting their balls, are used to being pushed.

Even today, I can only assume that sports for girls just aren't as intense—even though things are changing. The excuses I hear! "I just got my period!" "I'm tired!" "I don't want to sweat and mess up my hair/makeup/nails." Puh-leeze! They're just used to getting away with more.

Of course, not all women are like that. Some are game, no matter what. One woman I worked with was about three-quarters through her first Power Surge session when she looked up at me sweetly, and asked me if she was "supposed" to feel nauseated and ready to pass out! "Don't worry," I told her, "it will pass." And it did. It always does.

We're Just Warming Up!

All through Power Surge I like to tell my clients that we're just warming up. Some say, "What the hell am I warming up for? I'm not going to the Olympics!" This has become something of a personal joke with me because I like to think that they *can* go to the Olympics if they want to!

In fact, I never tell clients how much exercise we're really going to do because some of them probably would faint. If I told clients we were going to do a fifty-minute "warm-up" followed by a six-mile walk, followed by thirty minutes on a treadmill to get a really hot sweaty feeling, they'd look at me like I was out of my mind!

But at the end of the first day, and every day thereafter, my methods are borne out. Most times, their eyes are brighter, their smiles wider, their hips thinner, and they're a hell of a lot stronger than they ever imagined. I see this happen *all the time,* most recently with one of my adorable new clients, a twenty-eight-year-old pop music artist, originally from the Midwest, whose first single just hit *Billboard*'s Top 100 chart. She's pretty and well proportioned, with just ten extra pounds that really need to go. Like I told her—girls today want to be **F@#!*ING FIERCE!**

Our first workout was my regular Power Surge session, followed by a six-mile walk in Central Park, followed by a stretch and relaxing in a steam room (no wonder she feels that after just two sessions her body is changing!). But all along, I've been telling her that she can do much more than she thinks she can!

After her producers hired me, this client was excited to meet me because she had heard so much about me—but she was nervous. She said she was surprised at how down-to-earth I seemed; she didn't expect that at all! But even though I may run with the rich and famous, I come from the Midwest—a small town, Lorain, Ohio. I don't take the rich and famous . . . or what I call the "oh, dahling" set . . . or me all that seriously! People are people. It's all just a big game that I've learned how to play well. I really want more in my life than what I call air-kissing friends.

No Time to Exercise? I Don't Think So!

They say that people should exercise at least three times a week for a minimum of twenty minutes each time. Well, I always wondered who the f@#!* "they" were. Are they the same people who say pasta isn't fattening? Or that there's no such thing as cellulite? I say we should take a good hard look at how much of our behavior is influenced by "them" and figure out just who they are!

To me, asking how many times a week you should work out is like asking how many times a week you should brush your teeth or wash your face, shower or put on makeup. It just doesn't compute! I want working out to become part of your grooming, part of your life.

My answer is simple—*every day,* people! Every day! Just like a shower. Just like putting on makeup. It's not hard when you find some activity that you like—Rollerblading, running, jumping rope, tennis. Claudia Cohen, who does Regis and Kathie Lee's celebrity gossip segments, was one of my clients years ago—before she married (and ultimately divorced) Revlon CEO Ron Perelman. She loved skipping better than walking or jogging. We used to skip all around the huge rooms in her apartment—across the living room and around and around the dining room! To music, of course! This happens to be one of my favorite activities too.

Do whatever works best for you. Get creative—how about trying a trampoline? Recently, when I was in the Hamptons with one of my favorite clients, we stumbled on a trampoline at the stable where we were riding (it was meant to entertain the children while they were waiting for their riding lessons). Well, these big children put that trampoline to use—and my client and I liked it so much that she ended up buying one. She actually bought a full-sized trampoline; there are small ones you can buy for your home too. One top editor I know gets up a five A.M. to fit in an exercise hour. Her staff thinks she's crazy; she's not—because it's necessary! You make time for anything that is important—and your health and your body are important!

Are mornings too hectic for you (getting to an early class, or getting your kids to school and then to work yourself)? Well, every part of your life (and everyone else's) is hectic too. It's good to get exercise over with in the morning, but frankly I'd be satisfied wherever you find the time. If, like some women, you stick to a healthy diet during the day and lose control in the evenings, working out after work might be a solution for you, so you don't have so much unstructured evening time.

Okay, okay, some days you might have a perfectly good reason why a workout just won't work out—catching a transatlantic flight, maybe? But most times I just don't buy it. You're still going to shower, right? Well, I want your workout to be as automatic and as much a part of your life as a shower in the morning. This is body maintenance! This is health! This is not something expendable!

And I can be reasonable—if there *is* that day when it's totally impossible. Well, how about all those other days?

Every Excuse in the Book

I've probably heard every excuse in the book and then some about having no time to exercise. And, as I've also said before, I want you to make the time! Schedule an appointment with yourself—and don't cancel (even fifteen minutes is better than nothing!). *Just get the habit.* One woman had her secretary book her workout with me under a false name so that no one in the office knew where she was going; they only knew it was an uncancelable appointment! I guess she felt funny putting "High Voltage" in her daily calendar! Not to mention explaining to her personal secretary who—or what—High Voltage was! After this book, well, the secret weapon (as I have been called) will be out!

Over the years, I've heard it all. Here are some of the most common excuses. Which one is you?

● *I can't stick with it.*

Don't pooh-pooh me for stressing the music factor again, but music is the prime motivator. If you can't stick to working out, I can almost guarantee that you're not working out to music that you love. I had one client, a *Vogue* editor—a total doll!—who was known for her cool reserve. When I found a particular dance tape for her, though, that reserve melted away: it was so exciting for me to see her so into it: whooing and dancing away! I actually made up a dance step that I did at my energy concerts and called it "the Preston" after her!

Another very conservative client of mine, from a big pharmaceuticals family, couldn't stay with his exercise program until, much to my surprise, I found that Donna Summer's old disco classics turned him on! Then, once he got into the High Voltage high, he even began doing a fabulous free-style disco routine! I must say, even though I've seen this happen many times, it's still a thrill for me to see that kind of breakthrough. I live for it!

I also want you to look to your family and friends for support; let them know what your goals are, ask them to help you (and better yet, ask them to join you!). Fight boredom by taking a different walking route, trying a new video, or working out with a partner. If you're already working out to music, up the intensity—make it faster or stronger. In the health clubs, you often see people on treadmills or StairMasters who are watching TV or reading. As far as I am concerned, if they can read or watch TV, they're not pushing hard enough to get anywhere near that endorphin high I'm talking about. When you're pushing, you enter a zone that's almost like a meditative state. (P.S. That's how I meditate. And the feeling I get from this is what saved my ass!)

Finally, if your life is such a rat race that there truly isn't a minute to spare for yourself—let alone an hour—then something's got to give, something is drastically wrong, and you've got to seriously look into changing the pace of your life. My favorite response to clients who tell me about the rat race is, "And if you win, are you the best rat?" Hmmmmm. Good question, don't you think?

● *I'm too tired.*

Are you more awake in the morning? Or do you get your second wind in the early evening? Exercise any time of the day that you feel most energetic. You know your own body clock—and schedule—best.

I also tell my clients that during the first few days of working out, not only are you not going to be energized, you'll probably be exhausted. But working out is like climbing a hill. Once you reach the top of that hill, you will start to experience a high that takes you higher than any drug or stimulant or any other man-made substance can.

● *I'm a klutz.*

Maybe. Who am I to say that you're not? But—that doesn't mean you can't still be active. The answer for you may be walking. Long walks with your kids. Long walks around your block. Speed walks in the local park. Or try doing step aerobics (if you can climb stairs, you can do step!). One of my clients, Laura, a beautiful blonde who owns one of the biggest recording studios in New York City, and happens to be one of my most long-standing, adorable, and dearest clients, always says she is the world's biggest klutz! And she may be right! We laugh about this all the time, but after years of working with me, she still doesn't know the basic workout moves to Power Surge!

But I got Laura a step to do step aerobics and worked out the most basic up-and-down routine for her. We kid around that when I do a video, we're going to put in her routine for all the klutzes out there. Of course, she is the best-dressed—and now the fittest—klutz around!

● *I'm embarrassed to go to a gym and I can't afford a home trainer or fancy equipment.*

So you don't have a treadmill or StairMaster or bike at home. Most people don't. So march in place—that's aerobic. Do jumping jacks. Get a step. Skip. Put on music and dance (while you're doing your daily chores). Climb stairs (to the basement and back)—it's better than a StairMaster. Best of all, walk around the block. You don't have to go to a gym. *There is no excuse!*

Keep Your Workout Challenging

I also want you to challenge yourself with your workout: keep it fluid, keep it changing, set new goals. This might mean working out for an extra ten minutes, swimming or running an extra lap, picking up the pace of the music to something faster. For one client, during a step routine, I changed the beat of the music from time to time; for another we would take a different route on our daily walks.

I always recommend that clients get out and do a real walk, a real bike ride, go up and down real stairs, instead of just working out on equipment. Not even I could get someone to walk six miles on a treadmill during their very first workout—although I can certainly get them to do it outside, preferably on the beach, in the woods, in a park, or anywhere they can feel close to nature. If the weather is bad, I suggest they do what a lot of people do and walk in the mall—but no window-shopping please, and stay away from those fast-food nightmares.

The **Power Surge Workout**

This workout is designed for overall body conditioning. For best results, when you need a recharge, do the complete Power Surge Workout every day (it's not a requirement, but it is a goal). If, as with most people, time is a problem, try to fit in part of it—the ten-minute stretches, or the floor work, or the upper-body workout—a few times a week as a supplement to your daily dose of aerobic activity (that, people, is nonnegotiable!).

If your legs are already strong, for increased weight resistance, add ankle weights during your leg lifts, or hold your dumbbells while you're doing your squats and lunges. Depending on your pace and strength, the entire workout should take fifty-five minutes to an hour. And of course, these exercises won't bulk up your muscles because the emphasis is on multiple repetitions, not on pumping heavy weights. Dumbbells should be two, three, five, eight, or ten pounds each.

Volt-Note!

In some of these exercises (especially the crunches) you will notice that I have turned my head to the side and am smiling at the camera! I can't help it—if there's a camera around I'm going to smile. Like I say, I don't eat ham, I am one! You, however, may be more comfortable keeping your head straight.

Power Surge is based on classic fitness movements that many of you will already know. Therefore, it is not unfamiliar, gimmicky, or hard to remember. The **POWER** in Power Surge comes from the combination of these exercises, the balance with which they're put together (working every part of your body), and **YOU!** Remember to exhale as you are working your muscles and inhale when you return to your start position.

Part I:

Stretch and Flexibility (10 minutes)

Basic Pliés (Deep Knee Bends)

Stand straight, feet slightly apart, knees bent, so that your toes are turned out and your heels are in line with your shoulders. Bring your hands in front of you with your elbows slightly bent, fingers pointing toward the ground. Raise your hands over your head while at the same time straightening your knees. Return to start position.

Repeat 10 times.

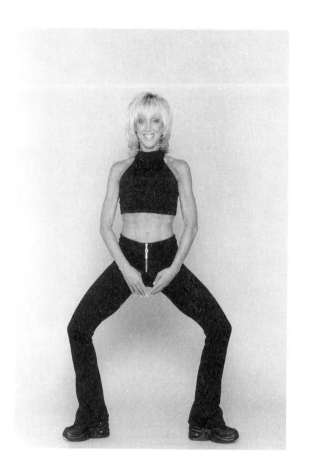
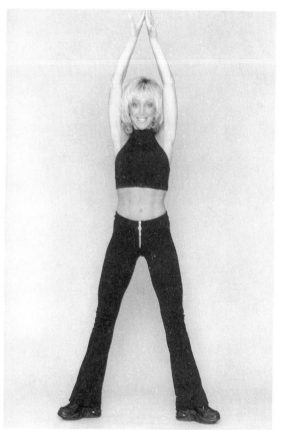

Opposite-Arm Stretches

Stand straight, feet slightly apart, a small bend in the knees. Bring your right arm up so that there is a 90-degree bend in your elbow, hand pointed toward the ceiling. Your left arm is in a relaxed position in front of your body. Bring your right arm up and over your head, bending your torso slightly to the left. Return to start position.

Repeat 10 times on each side.

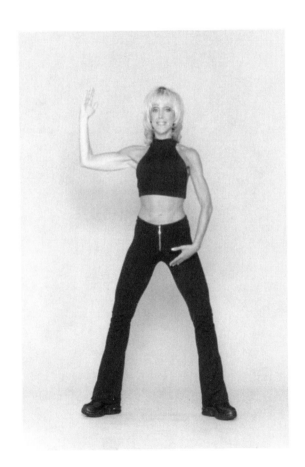
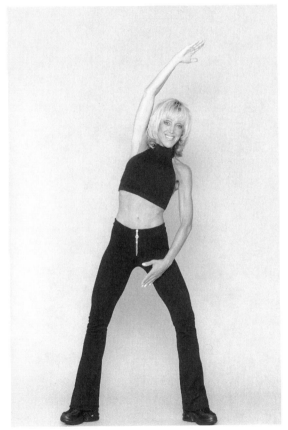

Windmill Stretches

Stand straight, feet slightly apart, a small bend in the knees. Your hands are in front of you, a slight bend in the elbows, fingers pointed toward the ground. Make a circle in front of your body, raising your arms as high as you can overhead. *Do 10 times, then reverse direction and repeat.*

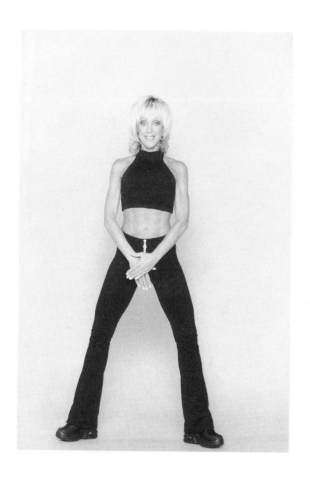 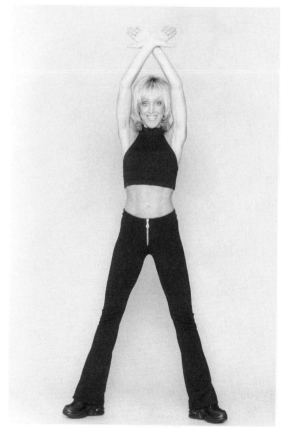

Side Toe Stretches

Stand straight, feet slightly apart, a small bend in the knees, arms reaching overhead. Bending at the waist, reach toward your right toes (or as far as you can go). Return to start position.

Alternate 3 times on each side.

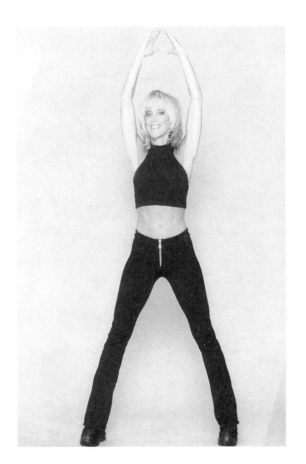 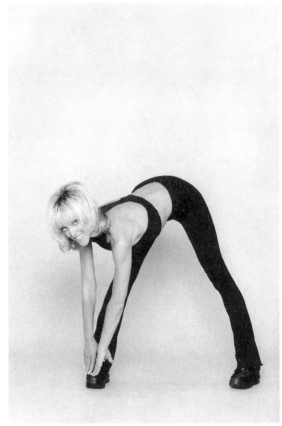

Bend-and-Stretches

Stand with your legs far enough apart, knees bent, so that you can put your hands on the ground in front of you. Straighten your knees and raise your butt toward the ceiling. Return to start position.

Repeat 5 times.

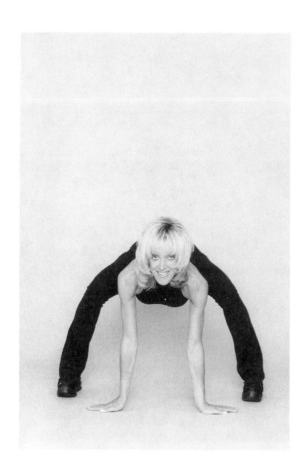
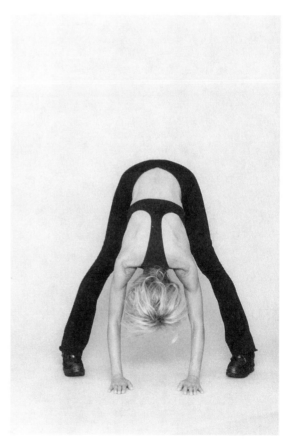

Neck Stretch

Stand straight, feet slightly apart, a small bend in the knees. Arms are loosely in front of you. Drop your chin to your chest. Hold for 2 counts and feel the stretch. Raise your chin to the ceiling. Hold and feel the stretch. Return to start position. *Repeat 3 times.*

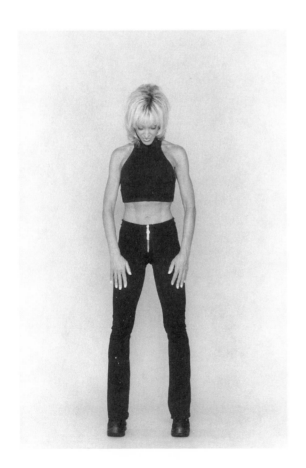 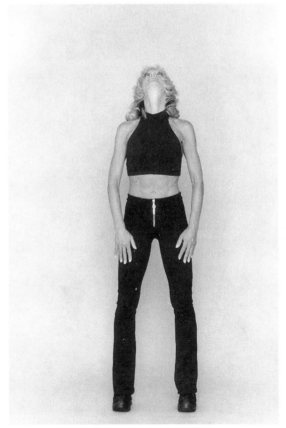

Head Rolls

Tilt your head to the right as if you were trying to put your ear on your shoulder. Repeat on the left. Turn your head to the left, looking out over your shoulder. Repeat on the right. Now, roll your head from shoulder to shoulder, keeping your chin toward your chest.

Repeat sequence 3 times.

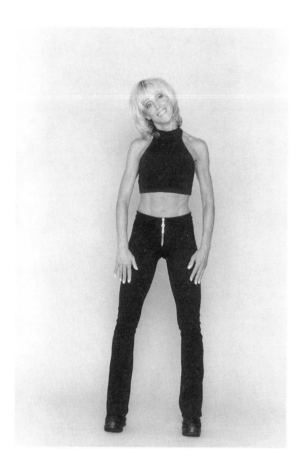
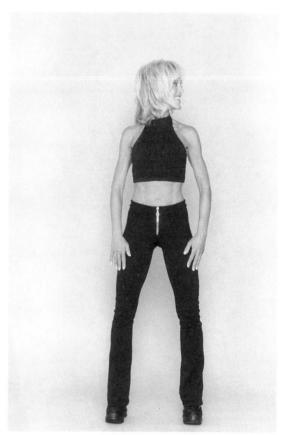

Shoulder Rolls

Stand straight, feet slightly apart, a small bend in the knees. Arms are relaxed at your sides. Contract your shoulders forward, roll them up toward your ears, and then as far behind you as you can go. Think of drawing a circle on a wall beside you.

Alternate rolling backward and forward 10 times.

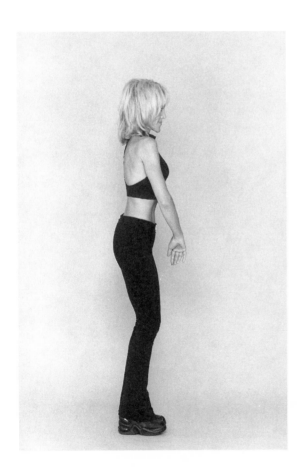

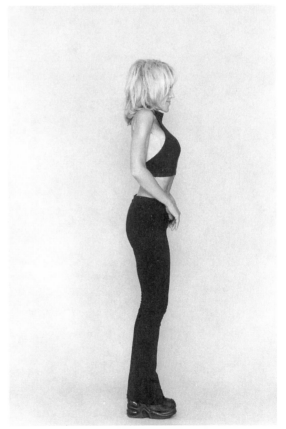

Power Twist Punches

Stand straight, feet slightly apart, a small bend in the knees. Arms are raised parallel to the floor, fists at chest level. With your right arm punch forcefully to your left while twisting slightly at the waist. Return to start position.
Do 3 sets of 10 on each side.

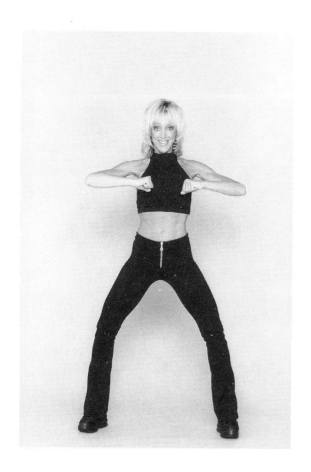
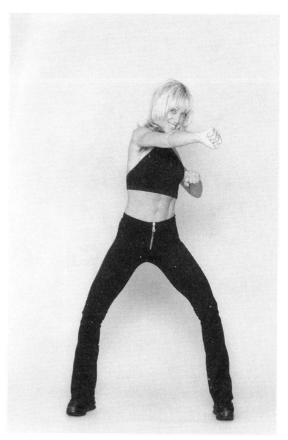

Part II:

Floor Work (20 minutes)

Forward Toe-Touch Stretches

Sit on the floor, legs together in front of you, feet flexed. Arms are raised high overhead. Reach forward as far as you can toward your toes. Keep your back as flat as possible. Return to start position.
Repeat 10 times.

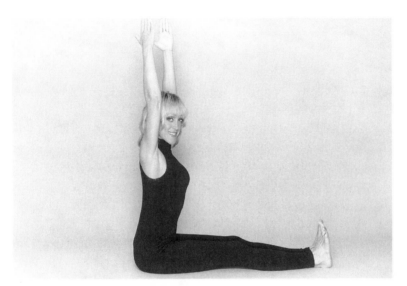

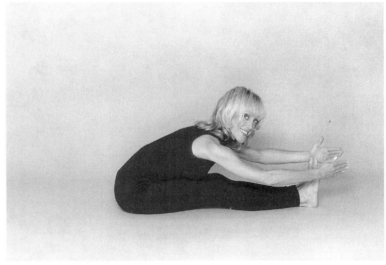

144

Side Stretches

Sit on the floor, legs as far apart as you can stretch comfortably. Arms are overhead. Turn at the waist to the right and reach for your toes. Hold to the count of 10. Return to start position. Repeat on left.

Do 3 times on each side.

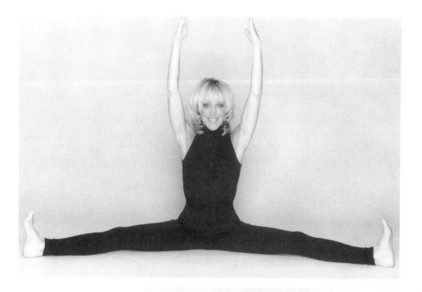

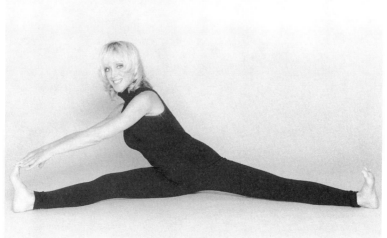

Yoga Stretches

Sit on the floor, knees bent, soles of your feet pressed together, hands holding your feet. Drop forward from the waist. Hold to feel the stretch. Don't bounce! Return to start position.

Repeat 3 times.

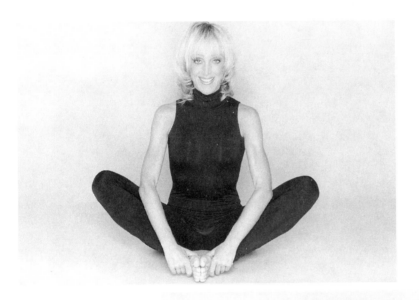

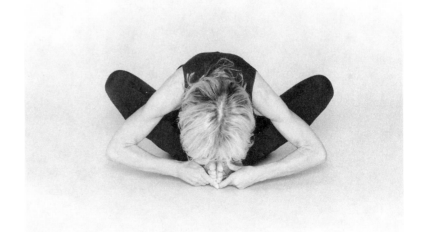

Ski-Style Warm-ups (ankle weights optional)

Sit on the floor, legs together in front of you, feet flexed. Arms are at your sides, hands supporting you on the floor. Keeping your right leg straight, lift your right foot off the floor about 6 inches; then lower it. Repeat 10 times. Then raise right leg and hold for a count of 10. Lower right leg and repeat with left leg. *Do 3 times for each leg.*

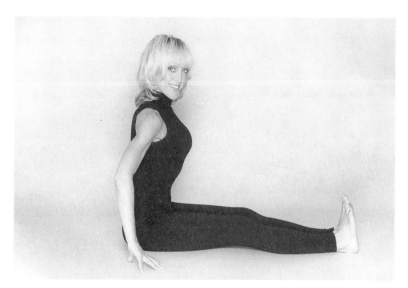

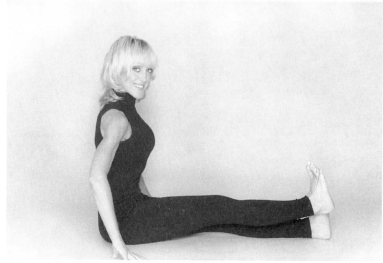

147

Rack Stretches

Lie on your back, arms overhead in a relaxed position. Reach as far as you can with your arms, and with feet flexed push with your heels.
Relax and repeat 3 times.

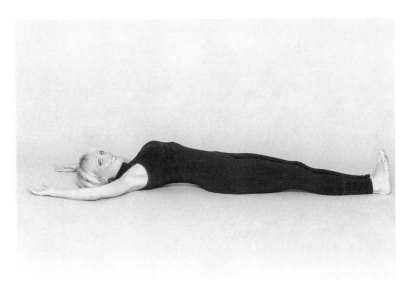

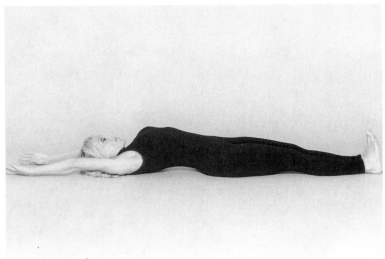

Leg Lifts

Lie on the floor, arms at sides, palms down. Left leg is bent with foot on the floor. Lift right leg, foot flexed, about 6 inches off the floor. Raise right leg toward the ceiling as high as you can go without straining. Return to start position. *Repeat 10 times on each leg.*

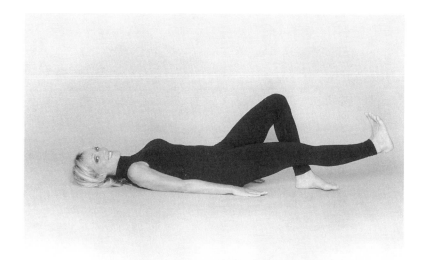

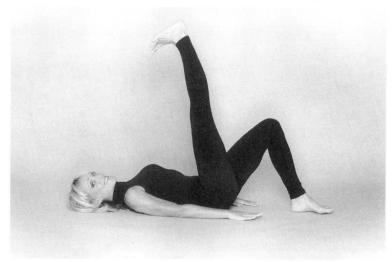

149

Oblique Side Crunches

Lie on the floor, hands behind head. Left leg is bent with foot on the floor. Right leg is bent with ankle resting on left knee. Lift your head, neck, and shoulders off the floor while at the same time twisting your waist so that your left elbow points toward your right knee. Return to start position.

Switch legs and repeat on the other side. Start at 20 reps and work up to 50—or more.

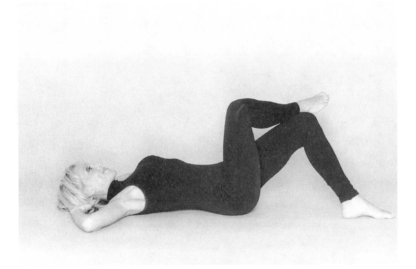

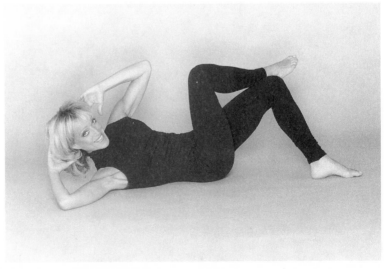

Chin-up Ab Crunches

Lie on the floor, hands behind head. Knees are bent and both feet are on the floor. Lift your chin, neck, and shoulders toward the ceiling. This is a small movement. To maintain proper position, imagine you are holding an orange under your chin. Return to start position.

Start at 20 reps and work up to 50—or more.

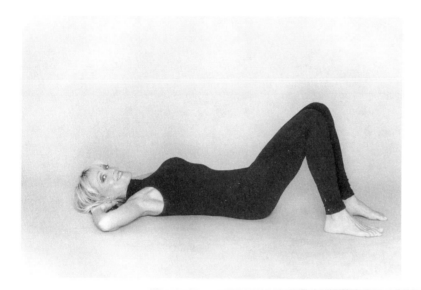

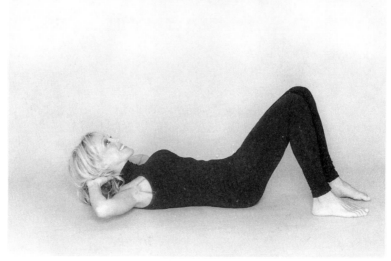

151

Crunches

Lie on the floor with hands on top of your head, elbows toward the ceiling. Knees are bent toward abs, lower legs point toward the ceiling with feet crossed. Contract your abs and bring your elbows and knees together by lifting your upper body off the floor. Return to start position.
Start at 20 reps and work up to 50—or more.

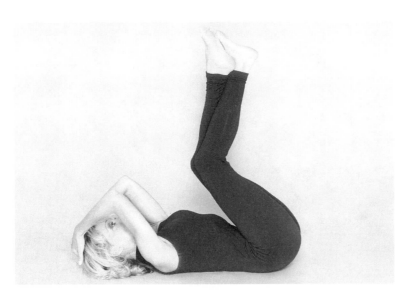

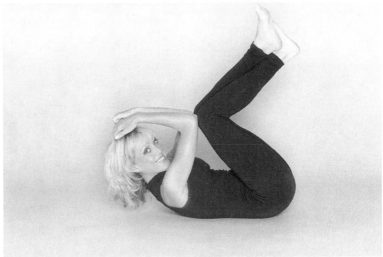

Lower Ab Lifts

Lie flat on the floor with arms at your sides, palms down. Lift your legs at a 90-degree angle with knees slightly bent and feet crossed. Lift your butt off the floor—feel it in your lower abs. Don't use your arms to push up. Return to start position.

Start at 20 reps and work up to 50—or more.

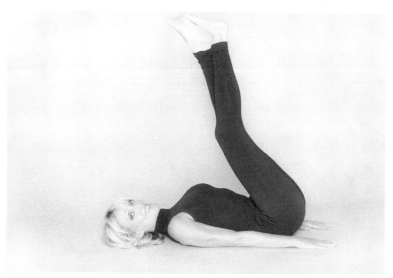

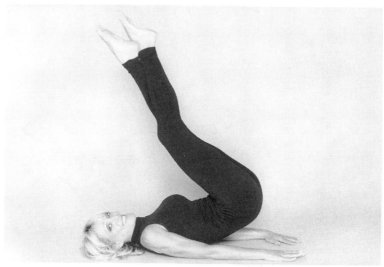

153

Butt Squeezes

Lie flat on the floor with arms at your sides, palms down. Knees are bent with feet on the floor. Lift your butt off the floor while contracting your butt muscles. Return to start position.

Start at 20 reps and work up to 50—or more.

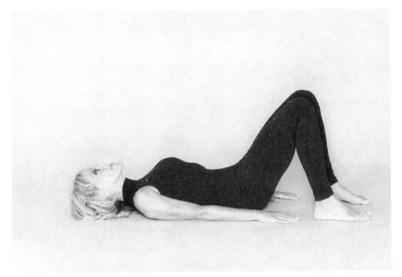

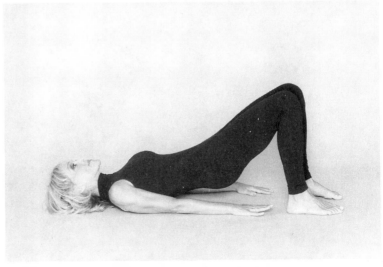

154

Outer-Thigh Lifts

Lie on your right side on the floor, right arm supporting your head, left arm in front of you for balance. Head, hips, and feet should all be aligned. Raise your left leg from the hip, with foot flexed, toward the ceiling. Keep hips parallel. Return to start position.

Start at 10 reps and work up to 50. Repeat on opposite side.

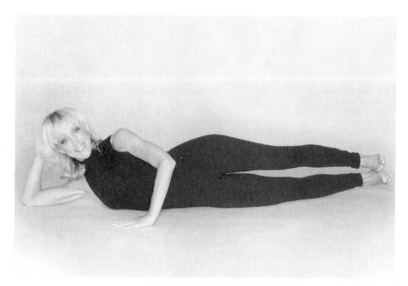

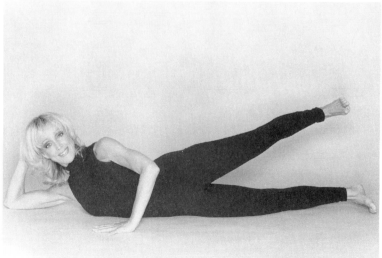

155

Inner-Thigh Lifts

Lie on your right side on the floor, right arm supporting your head, left arm in front of you for balance. With your left knee bent drop your left leg forward so that your lower left leg is resting on the floor in front of you. Keep your hips aligned and pointed toward the ceiling. With foot flexed, raise your right leg toward the ceiling. Return to start position.

Start at 10 reps and work up to 50. Repeat on opposite side.

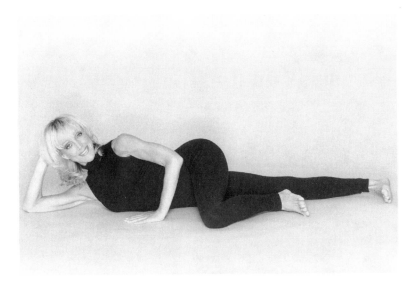

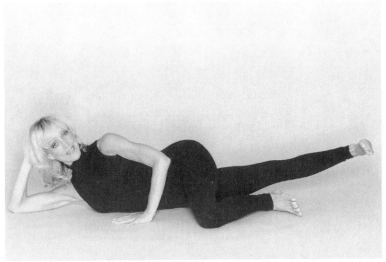

Butt Lifts

Rest your forearms and right knee on the floor. With your left knee bent, raise left leg so that your thigh is parallel to the floor and the bottom of your foot is toward the ceiling. Raise your left foot as though you want to put a footprint on the ceiling. Keep your hips forward. Return to start position.
Repeat on opposite side. Start with 10. Work up to 50 on each side.

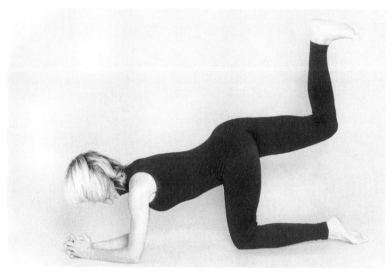

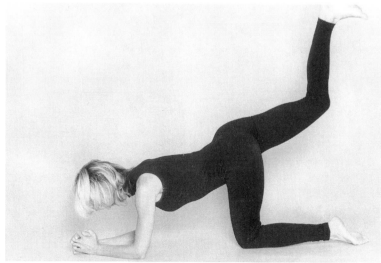

Push-ups

These modified push-ups are included for all levels. Feel free to do military-style push-ups (with feet extended behind you) like I usually do. Kneel on the floor with feet lifted and crossed behind you. Arms are straight and hands are on the floor slightly wider than your shoulders. Lower your body, bending your elbows out to the sides. Return to start position.

In the beginning, do as many as you can; work up to 3 sets of 20.

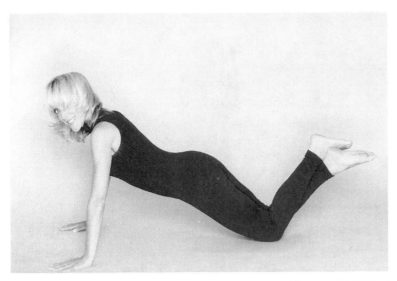

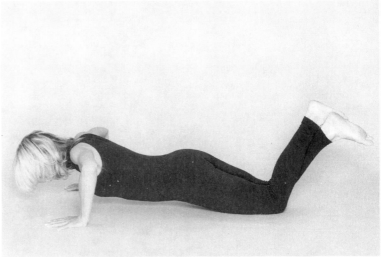

Angry Cat Stretches

Kneel on the floor, arms straight, with hands on the floor slightly wider than your shoulders. Keep your back flat. Contract your abs toward the ceiling while arching your back and dropping your head slightly forward. Return to start position. *Repeat 10 times.*

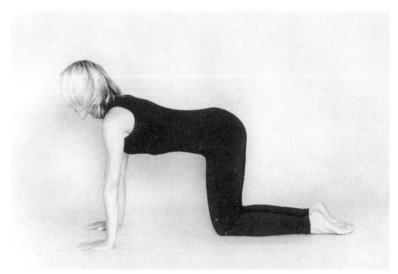

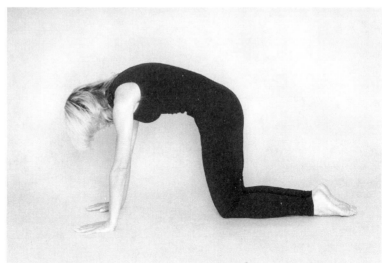

159

Floor Stretch

Lie on the floor, knees bent toward your chest, hands reaching toward your feet. Pull your feet into your chest while raising your head off the floor. Chin reaches toward knees.

Hold for a count of 10.

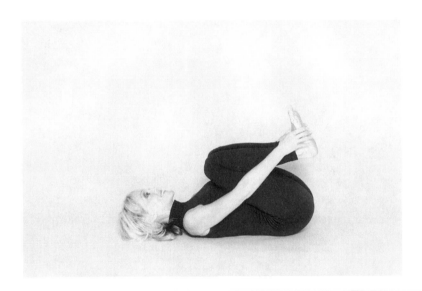

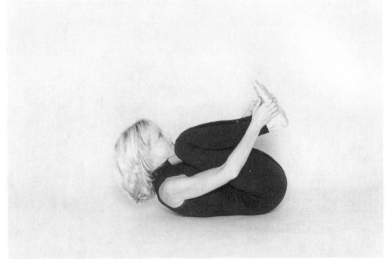

Squats

Stand straight, feet slightly apart, a small bend in the knees. Arms are relaxed at your sides. (Optional—as shown—hold a weight in each hand.) Keeping your back straight, bend your knees as if you are going to sit down in a chair. Make sure your butt doesn't drop below your knees. As you return to start position, squeeze your butt.

Start with 10. Work up to 3 sets of 20.

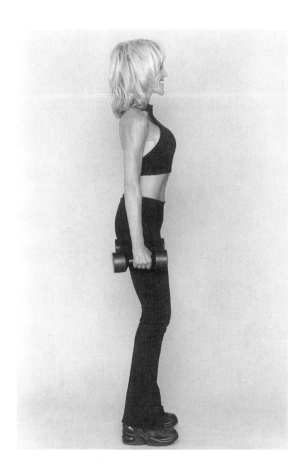
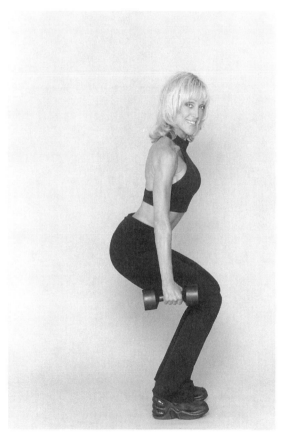

Lunges

Stand straight, feet slightly apart, a small bend in the knees. Arms are relaxed at your sides. (Optional—as shown—hold a weight in each hand.) Take a step forward onto your right leg so that your right thigh is parallel to the floor. Drop your left knee toward the floor while raising your left heel. As you return to start position, squeeze your butt.

Start with 10. Work up to 3 sets of 20.

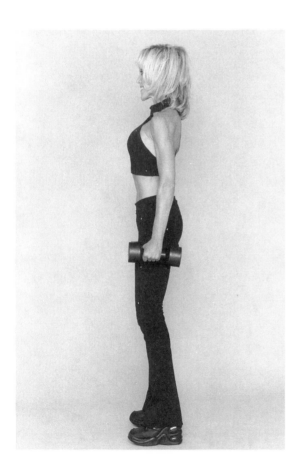
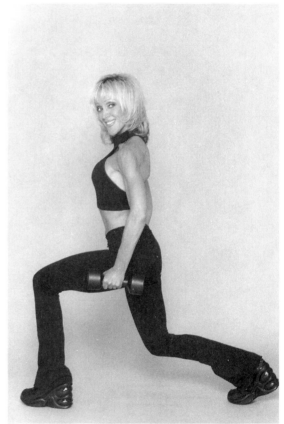

Calf Raises

Stand straight, feet together, arms relaxed at your sides. Lift up on your toes. Return to start position.

Start with 3 sets of 10. Work up to 3 sets of 20.

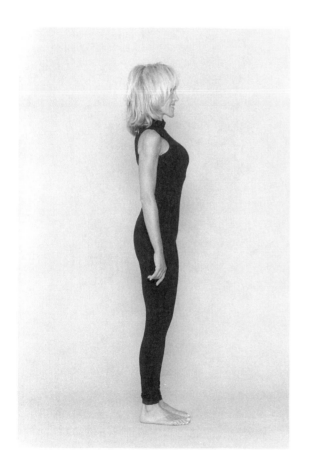
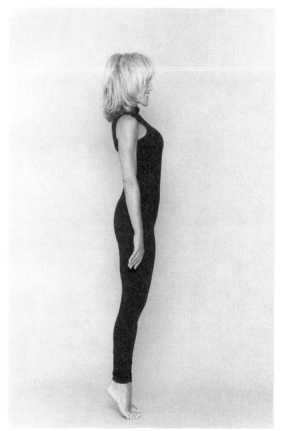

Part III:

Upper-Body Workout with Weights
(10 minutes)

Biceps Curls

Stand straight, feet together, knees slightly bent, arms at your sides with a weight in each hand, palms forward. Bend your right elbow, keeping it at your side, and raise your right hand toward your shoulder. Lower your right hand and raise your left hand toward your left shoulder.

This is 1 rep. Repeat 15 times, alternating hands.

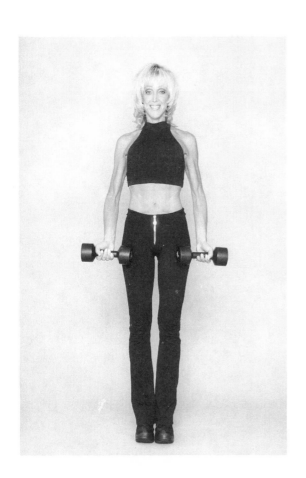
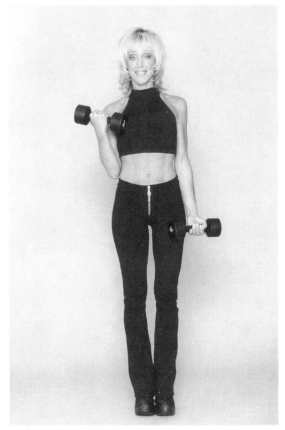

Lateral Lifts

Stand straight, feet together, knees slightly bent, arms at your sides with a weight in each hand, palms facing thighs. Raise your right arm directly in front of you to chest height, keeping your elbow slightly bent. Lower your right arm and raise your left arm directly in front of you to chest height.
This is 1 rep. Repeat 15 times, alternating hands.

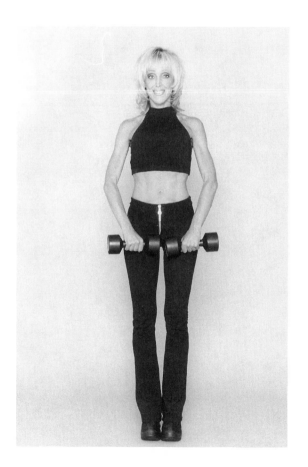
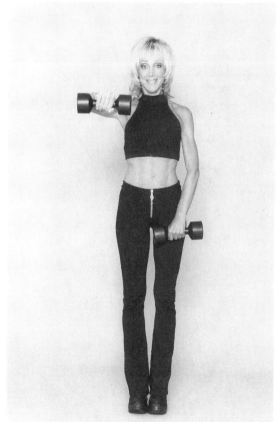

Shoulder Lifts

Stand straight, feet together, knees slightly bent, both arms raised so that your elbows are bent and your hands, holding weights, are toward the ceiling. Extend your arms up so that the weights meet over your head. Return to start position. *Repeat 15 times.*

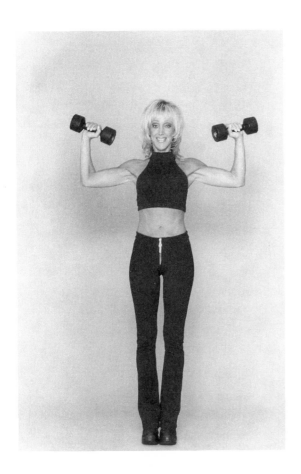 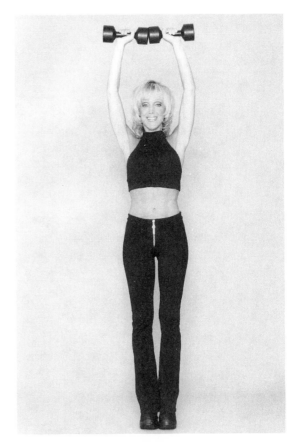

166

Deltoid Lifts

Stand straight, feet together, knees slightly bent, arms bent so that your hands, holding weights, meet in front of your lower abs. Raise your elbows to the sides, keeping elbows bent, arms parallel to the floor, and the back of your hands toward the ceiling. Return to start position.
Repeat 15 times.

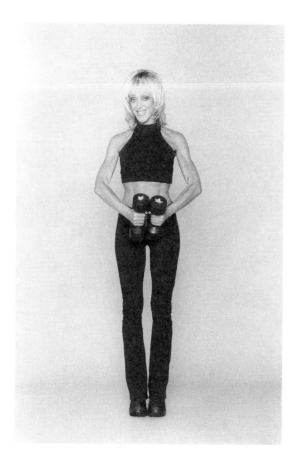 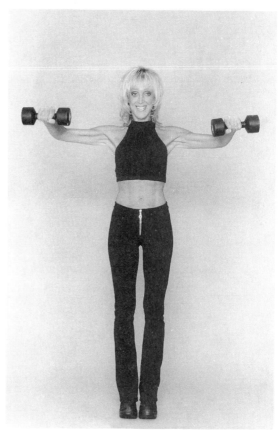

Triceps Hammers

Stand straight, knees slightly bent. Hold one weight in both hands, with arms extended over your head. Bend your elbows, keeping them close to your ears, and dip the weight behind your head. Return to start position.
Repeat 15 times.

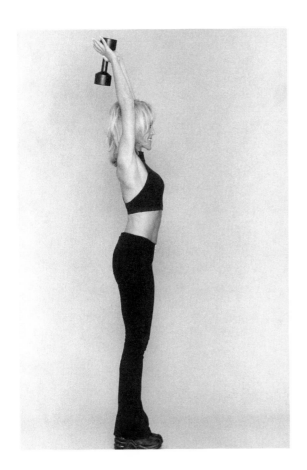 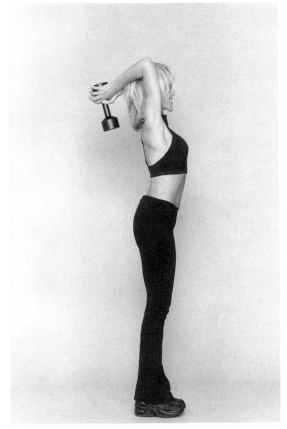

Part IV: 20 Minutes of Kick-Ass Aerobics

Choose from treadmill, StairMaster, jumping rope, biking, stair climbing, walking uphill, swimming, etc., followed by a cool-down stretch.

Part V: Whoo!

Inhale 3 times, gather all your energy, and say:

One, two, three, Energy UP! Whoo!
Energy UP! Whoo!
Kiss, Kiss [on each side]

This is very important. Doing the "Whoo!" gives you an energy jolt, which is a great way to end your exercise routine—if this doesn't happen you've been doing a routine designed by a Voltage impostor!

The Cellulite Sellout

Exercise will not get rid of cellulite (which, trust me, does exist, contrary to what many doctors are still saying). And you can be thin and still have cellulite—I know because I have it. One of the cool things about being fifty is that I can admit to having cellulite (I blame it on my age—but I bet I'd have a ton more if I ate flour and salt!). But hello! I've had it since I was fourteen—as do *all* the women in my family—and quite a few of the top models I've met.

Now I don't have a lot of cellulite, by any means. My ex-husband used to say that I spent thousands of dollars getting rid of cellulite that no one could see but me. I think I went to every expensive cellulite-removal program in town (and of course, remember that my sister and I ran our own cellulite business—so I know what I am talking about!).

Exercise will not get rid of cellulite. Take flour, sugar, and salt out of your diet and your cellulite will go down dramatically. This was something I first became aware of when I was at Duke University with my husband. On a no-salt diet, my rings started to become loose (I actually went down half a ring size!). And once I eliminated flour in addition to the salt, I saw my cellulite almost melt away.

The Plastic Surgery Option

Sometimes, not even exercise (not even my workout!) can do it all—which is why I'm obviously a big believer in plastic surgery. When I say this is what fifty looks like, I mean that for me, this is what fifty looks like with a lot of work done! If you are interested in plastic surgery and haven't had any before, I advise meeting with no more and no less than three board-certified surgeons for whom you have personal recommendations (otherwise you'll drive yourself nuts!). Luckily for me, I knew the girlfriend of my first plastic surgeon, so I made sure he got to bed early the night before my surgery (not a bad idea if you can swing it!). The other day, I actually had two of my favorite clients recuperating from nose jobs at my home at the same time, complete with a private nurse. Let me tell you, this was a three-ring circus and a slumber party with nose bandages, all rolled into one! But we pulled them through!

Aging

As far as age goes, I've always gone with the old saying that you're only as old as you feel. I've seen energetic sixty-year-olds, and schlumpy nineteen-year-olds—so for me, age is a nonissue in terms of health and fitness level. As you age, you become smarter, more experienced—and you should be getting stronger, not weaker. I want aging to be something we all embrace (after all, it's a passage we all have to make, so we may as well embrace it). As that popular new TV commercial says, it's not just about adding years to your life, it's about adding life to your years! (The product is loaded with sodium, but the commercial is right on the money!)

As for people becoming more injury-prone as they age, part of the reason for that is because often they haven't been stretching and working out. If that's where you're starting from, I'll take that into consideration, of course, but that's not where we're going! We're going to the **Volt**-Age, where you get leaner and meaner as you get older. I'm proof of that! My generation said don't trust anyone over thirty. Well, we're way over thirty, and we're changing the rules again!

Remember, No Excuses

Finally, I want to remind you, once again, that I've heard every excuse there is for not fitting exercise into your life—and I don't buy into it! It's *non-negotiable*, people, and there's no middle road here. Lack of time? Time isn't the real issue; it's making the workout a priority (hey, if someone was paying you to work out, I guarantee you'd find the time!). What's the use of a fast-paced creative job if it's killing you? If you can't fit my Power Surge into your life, then I'm telling you right now, you've got to change your life.

Remember, with Power Surge, you don't need special clothes, an expensive health club membership, or a ton of equipment in order to work out. You don't need to have worked out before, and you don't need to be especially athletic or even coordinated. You do need the commitment and you do need to make it a habit—to set aside the time each and every day. If on some days, you just can't squeeze in that Power Surge hour, do it for a half hour (more is better, but some is better than none). Be creative with your time too. One of my clients lifts weights while listening to the evening news.

If you do, I guarantee the rewards will be worth it. Sure, the workout will strengthen your body and speed your weight loss by increasing your body's metabolism (what was hard will get easier; what was tight will fit). But more important, working out is a step toward taking charge of your life: it's a step toward stress control and self-esteem, a defense against heart disease, osteoporosis, fatigue, and burnout. There are twenty-four hours in the day, people. Set aside just one of those hours for your workout and it'll make the others worthwhile.

ENERGY UP! WHOO!

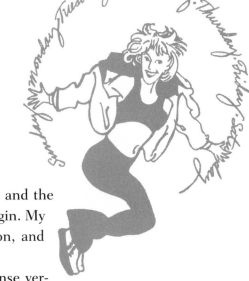

Chapter 7

COUNTDOWN TO SPA WEEK— READY, SET, ENERGY UP!

Now that you've got the Star Power Plan and the Power Surge Workout, you're ready to begin. My Star is not to wish upon, it's to act upon, and that's what this chapter is all about.

Spa Week is a slightly more intense version of my Star Power Plan combined with the Power Surge Workout. For my clients, it's a week of commitment and transformation—changing old habits and developing new ones. We usually go away together; we eat only special **SPA WEEK** meals, prepared by my chef; we work out—*and I take charge.*

For you, Spa Week is the week where you take my program and get your body and mind used to High Voltage ways. I want you to follow it just as if I were at your side. There are specific dos and don'ts in terms of what you are going to eat (no artificial sweeteners on Spa Week, for example); there are specific activities—exercises, affirmations, beauty treatments— that you'll be required to do.

But all clients—and you too—have got to go through Spa Week to make the High Voltage transformation. At the end of Spa Week—just seven days—you will look and feel lighter and healthier, and be more energized than you've ever felt before.

Getting Ready for Spa Week

Before you begin your Spa Week, there are certain things you will need to do and prepare. Below is a "countdown" to Spa Week, with a special assignment for you to do every day.

In the countdown ahead, I'm going to explain each step in detail. But in general, you're going to use the week before your Spa Week to prepare yourself, mind and body, for your commitment to a new High Voltage way of living. You're going to remove foods with flour, sugar, and salt from your kitchen and replace them with choices that are healthy and Voltage-safe. You're going to spend some time figuring out when you're going to do your workout and mark down on your calendar the exact times you're going to be exercising (it's also a good idea to start getting more movement into your life now, so that Spa Week won't be such a shock to your system!). The same goes for Spa Week beauty treatments: I want you to use this time to block out time for beauty—and stock up on any creams, ingredients, or grooming aids you may need.

> ### Countdown to Spa Week
>
> Day 7   Keeping a Food Diary
> Day 6   Doing Your Kitchen CleanUp
> Day 5   Stocking the High Voltage Pantry
> Day 4   Preparing for the Power Surge Workout
> Day 3   Setting Up a Support System
> Day 2   Recharging Your Environment
> Day 1   Planning Your Beauty Regimen

Are you ready? Then, let's begin.

Seven Days Before Spa Week: Keeping a Food Diary

Before I take on new clients, I insist on their keeping a food diary to open their eyes (and mine) to exactly what their eating patterns have been. Are they living on processed foods? Are they grabbing sandwiches here and there? Half the time, my dears, people don't even know what they're eating. But that diary tells me all! It's a total reality check!

For example, the most frequent comment I get from potential clients is: "I just don't eat that much! I really don't know what the problem is." For some people, that may be true, but I'll tell you, most people are *amazed* at how much they end up writing down!

When clients tell me they don't eat much junk, I say, "Define junk." True, you may not be eating candy bars and Fritos, but I bet you eat bread and pizza and pasta. Remember, to me, junk is anything with white flour in it. So, think to yourself, Do I eat much white flour?

A food diary helps me to understand what is causing a client's problem with food. And since clients are paying through the nose for my time and opinions, you can bet that I usually end up getting an honest accounting. (Besides, if clients are not honest, who are they fooling but themselves?) Remember, when someone hires someone like me (actually, no one's like me!), it's because they genuinely **want to make change in their lives.** After all, I don't advertise. I don't go after people. Clients have to seek me out—and once they've gone to that trouble *and* agreed to my terms, they're ready to do things **MY WAY.** I ask for just one week of diary keeping, but many people find it such an effective tool, they keep it up long after the week is over.

Before **YOU** start my program I recommend that you keep a food diary too, ideally for a full week, but for at least three *typical* days to help discover your trigger foods. A day when you're on a business trip or vacation, going to the NBA playoffs, throwing your second cousin a baby shower, or attending your boss's twenty-fifth-anniversary party is *not* a typical day.

Then I want you to analyze the diary. Maybe, like some of my clients, your diary reads in a fairly healthy way for the morning and early afternoon, but you tend to indulge in junk as the afternoon and evening wear on. I can tell you right now, if you don't take time to eat right during the day, you'll go *berserk* in the evening (trust me: if you let yourself really get hungry, you **WILL** eat everything in sight!).

Maybe you're eating something that is simply wrong for your body and system. One top model I worked with who was naturally thin as a rail (she hired me for energy and flexibility!) never realized that flour was causing her energy drain. But her diary was the eye-opener: it turned out to be filled with high-flour junk she grabbed on shoots, such as crackers and cheese, bagels, tiny hors d'oeuvres slapped on crackers, and breadsticks.

Another client, a well-known recording star, told me she didn't know where her extra weight was coming from: she thought she was *already* eating in a High Voltage way. And she was . . . but not quite! This client was a vegetarian; she loved salads—which were, in fact, her mainstay—but her diary pinpointed the answer: all the sauces she put on her brown rice and vegetables and the dressings on her salads were a salt and high-calorie nightmare! Problem found; problem solved!

Most often, diaries reveal flour addictions. Sometimes I think this country lives on bagels for breakfast, sandwiches or pizza for lunch, and pasta for dinner! **DOUGH, DOUGH, DOUGH**—which simply turns into cellulite and fat!

But when clients have a weight problem, they're not at all conscious of what they're eating. It's a bite here, a bite there. After you start adding everything up, you have a long, long list! Plus, many clients really *don't* eat all that much, but they do most of their eating after six P.M., which can be a BIG problem. When you have your main meal at seven (plus snacks for the rest of the evening) and then go to sleep, your fuel isn't being used for anything but dreamtime. It's one bad habit I hope I can help you break—at least some of the time. You wonder why you wake up in the morning with puffy eyes, fingers, and ankles? Well, that's one reason!

Keeping a food diary is a device I use for convincing the occasional skeptic where he or she has gone astray.

For example, Wendy, thirty-five, a newspaper reporter whom I met when she was writing a story about me, was, like many journalists, a bit skeptical of my no flour, no sugar, no salt mandate, but she was willing to give the food diary a try. As I said before, *clients* are less resistant. They already come to me ready to play follow the leader, **MY** way!

Believing that her own diet was fairly healthy (and low in salt—a common misconception!), Wendy agreed to keep a food diary for a week—"as an experiment," she qualified—but just three days of entries immediately

Volt-Note!

A food diary is one of the tools I use to reinforce my system and keep my clients aware of what they're eating (that's why we even keep the diary on **SPA WEEK**). Does it make my clients think too much about food? Perhaps at first. But so many of them are obsessed about food and their weight to begin with. I'm about taking their obsession and trying to make it work for them, not against them!

told me why she was never able to lose the last ten pounds she had put on after the birth of her daughter, who was already five years old.

Wendy's food patterns were typical of many women who are trying to juggle home, family, and career. Even though she was obviously trying to eat in a healthy way, to me her entries practically screamed out loud with addictions to dough and hidden sugar and salt! I also noticed that as careful as she was when she started out in the mornings, as the day went on and she became more tired and stressed, her resolve and intentions deteriorated.

Any purse-sized notebook will do for your food diary (or you can even keep track on your home or office computer). Note: Ideally, I'd like you to keep up your diary during Spa Week too, and afterwards. Until High Voltage ways become second nature to you, I think you'll find it a terrific and effective tool.

Food Diary How-tos:

- Write down what you eat, the times you eat, and if possible, the circumstances (hey, if you always reach for a Reese's Peanut Butter Cup after talking to your boyfriend or your mother on the phone, chances are, it's a relationship-based energy block that you're feeding). One client of mine, a well-known photographer, had no problem sticking to a healthy diet when he was in his own studio. It was long days on location when the food was brought in by a catering company that slipped him up.

  Your food diary will also reveal significant eating patterns. For instance, if you consistently eat lunch or dinner on the late side, or skip meals, you may be letting yourself get too hungry, tired, or stressed before meals, and are more prone to overeat or make an unhealthy food choice that triggers a craving.

- Write down everything you put in your mouth, and as I say to some of the young single girls I work with, I do mean everything! Anything that goes in your mouth—and anything you swallow (this always gets a chuckle)! But seriously, I'm talking about the ravioli—or two—that you pop in your mouth when you're preparing your kids' dinner. That lick of your daughter's ice cream cone. The handful of M&M's you may absentmindedly scoop up in the office lounge. One client found her problem in her family's after-dinner cleanup ritual—and you may too. If you finish off your toddler's lamb chop when you're clearing the dinner dishes, along with the last of the kids' pasta, a quarter of a potato, and two spoons of chicken-flavored rice mix, it adds up.

● If you attend a party, I want a list of the hors d'oeuvres you nibble—those tiny time bombs add up too. And don't forget the salty peanuts you munch when you meet your office buddies for an after-work drink. Plus, "tastes" count too. The "taste" of chicken Parmesan from your date's plate (and don't forget the "bite" of his apple-walnut pie à la mode). The last of your girlfriend's cheeseburger here, a breadstick there. Come on, you're a grown-up—don't you know by now what a breadstick tastes like? You certainly know what it looks like on your thighs! "Tastes" only trigger cravings . . . they don't satisfy them. Better to steer clear and stay clean.

Six Days Before Spa Week: Doing Your Kitchen Cleanup

Another thing that my clients have to agree to before **SPA WEEK** is to let me come into their homes and clean out their kitchen cabinets. Let me tell you, this can be one dramatic event! But—it's another way that I get firsthand insight into their food habits.

Once I've launched an attack on an unsuspecting client's kitchen, I flatter myself that it's never quite the same. While I'm there, things fly! Flour, sugar, and salt—they've got to go! I swoop down. I sweep off the cabinet shelves. I empty the cupboards. At the top of my junk list are any packaged baked goods like Entenmann's—it's gotta go. I mean, if they're serious **IT'S GOTTA GO!** I dump out the refrigerator and freezer. And I admit it: this is fun. After a while, it's the rare client who doesn't start to giggle and get into the spirit!

One supertalented musician I worked with was a sucker for gourmet preserves—loaded with sugar!—and collected them from all over the world. We cleared his pantry of at least forty different flavors! Novelist Tama

Janowitz had a supply of cookies and easy-to-eat munchy foods (anything that was convenient to eat while she was writing). But out they went! Then there was that famous model who had a secret stash of Ring Dings! I found them under the paper towels and napkins. Gone! Poof!

I've never been surprised yet at a kitchen cleanup. In fact, what would surprise me is if I opened up the pantry and found really healthy food for a change. **THAT** would be a shocker. But I'm pretty hard to surprise when it comes to junk.

Still, model Beverly Peele's kitchen was one of worst I ever had to tackle. Even I found it hard to believe that this beauty with the exotic, almond-shaped eyes was fueling her body with Cheetos, Fritos, Oreos, Cookie Crisp cereal, Twinkies, and Chef Boyardee! I ended up carting away at least four industrial-sized garbage bags full of junk! The food was so bad, people, that I actually felt guilty donating it to a shelter!

RuPaul and I go way back, but we became especially close when he asked me to create High Voltage morning "Energy Breaks" for his fabulous radio show on WKTU—the first time a mainstream radio station has allowed anyone to send love and positive messages over the airwaves ("If you don't love yourself," he roars, "how the hell you gonna love anybody else!"). This is opposed to the negative rantings of someone like Howard Stern—who seems to have little use for women my age. Wouldn't you know that Howard, the self-proclaimed King of All Media, would be challenged by Ru, the self-proclaimed Queen! (And then, of course, there's me—the self-proclaimed Queen of Energy!)

Ru, who is one of the most special people on the planet—definitely in touch with his higher power!—was an immediate convert to my program. He's famous for his incredible body—and he wants to keep it that way.

When I went to the stunning West Village loft that Ru shares with his companion, George, I noticed that the kitchen counters seemed a *little* high, but I didn't pay much attention. Then I realized I could barely see the food in the cabinets. At first, I assumed that the kitchen cabinets had been *custom-designed* for their height—six four and six seven!—and I'm a lean, mean five four (the living room furniture seemed big to me too!). Then I realized that they simply kept all their food on the second and third shelves. So I just scrambled onto the counter and began clearing.

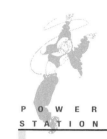

The basis for Ru's diet, by the way, was pasta and canned foods and vegetables—on the assumption that it all was fairly healthy, not being aware of the massive salt content. But between the soups, the prepackaged gravies, and your basic, salty cheeses, it was like a salt factory in there! In short order, we put together several large cartons to give away to the homeless. And he now has his meals prepared for him by a private chef, who delivers them weekly.

Michelle Visage, RuPaul's adorable co-host, has also taken my program to heart—and then some! She truly lives it. All it took was one supermarket trip with me and it just clicked for her.

After I hit my clients' cupboards, I ransack the refrigerator—a prime depository for condiments like barbecue sauce, pickles, cheeses, and those *dangerous* leftovers from take-out meals (I like to joke that I actually ex-or-cise them).

The bread box is usually another trouble spot (one client kept "emer-gency" cake mixes in hers!). As for most people—puh-leeze! Seasoned crou-tons, oily Chinese noodles, six different kinds of crackers, fudge cookies, pita crisps, minimuffins, and more. One of my clients did a precleaning for me—and, trying to be helpful, packed her bread and rolls away in the freezer. "What are you saving them for?" I asked her. "Expecting some company you don't like?" People, there's no need to hold on to this stuff for later—*unless you're planning to cheat, planning to backslide, not really willing to change your old eating patterns for new ones!*

Understandably, most clients are apprehensive about my High Volt-age kitchen cleanup. But it gets the point across, and it gets rid of potentially addictive foods that can tempt you into straying from my program (out of sight, out of mind, out of body, I say). The kitchen cleanup is especially im-portant in the first few months of my program, when clients are still form-ing new habits and it's easy to slip if the food is around.

One of my clients, Susanna, a highly successful clinical psychologist and mother of two, is a vibrant redhead of forty-five whose self-confidence was apparent the minute she walked in the room—as were the extra twenty-five pounds she had put on over the last few years as she was building her

179

therapy practice and teaching at a famous hospital. But she was raring to go: the minute I explained my program to her, it clicked! Like I said, you have to be ready to make a change! We quickly agreed that she would be this book's "kitchen cleanup" example.

Just two days after we met, I made my way to her beautiful Upper East Side townhouse to do my thing. Although many of my clients are single and live alone, Susanna is a working mom, and I had to consider her husband, as well as her son, age ten, and daughter, seven.

While my celebrity clients often have cooks (whom my chefs usually retrain in the High Voltage way), like most of us, Susanna does her own cooking. In fact, she's quite an accomplished hand in the kitchen. Her favorite way to relax from the pressures of her job is to prepare a big, casual dinner (then, usually pasta, garlic bread, and salad), for half a dozen friends! Unlike some people who complain to me, "Voltage, there's nothing to eat on your program," Susanna immediately saw dozens of possibilities for adapting her favorite recipes to my requirements (you'll find some of her ideas in our recipe section).

During our precleanup interview, I learned that Susanna's family ate a lot of healthy, steamed vegetables and fresh fruit, but they also ate a lot of starches and pasta. The first thing I did at her house was to clear off the specific pantry shelves that were going to be "hers." Then we went to work. (By now, I bet you already know the things that ring my **DANGER! HIGH VOLTAGE!** bell. I guess I owe the power supply plants something—all that free advertising!)

Here's Susanna's kitchen-cleanup scenario:

Out go the instant soups. Ditto for the linguine, fettucine, and elbow macaroni. The tuna packed in water stays. The Jell-O goes. Out with the condiments. Onto Susanna's shelf go the vanilla, the coffee, the herbal tea, and her collection of spices. The canned vegetables (corn and peas, packed with salt and sugar)—I don't think so! Rice cakes (the good ones—no salt) stay. The salsa—switch it for a no-salt version or make your own. Garbagey rice mixes—*forget about it*. Crackers, chips—out with it all! The honey—

maybe for later, when her weight is where she wants it. It can stay. The oatmeal stays; the applesauce goes (switch it for a version with no sugar added).

On to the refrigerator. Pasta salad with arugula—**OUT!** Rigatoni with sun-dried tomatoes and mozzarella—**OUT!** A bowl of hard-boiled eggs and a covered dish with fresh spinach seasoned with garlic and lemon juice—**VERY NICE**—they can stay. Out with the Dijon mustard and mayonnaise, out with the Parmesan cheese and the lemon-pear butter.

From the freezer: Mint chocolate chip ice cream goes. Lovely containers of homemade soups and curries (she assures me they have no salt) stay.

It was, Susanna admitted, a true whirlwind learning experience!

> **Volt-Note!**
>
> If, like Susanna, you and your family eat a lot of pasta and you're wondering about spinach, tomato, artichoke, and other "vegetable" pastas—well, don't! Baby, it's just the same old flour that someone waved a bunch of spinach over to give it some color. Please—I can't emphasize it enough—any of you women out there who have cellulite problems, any of you guys whose bodies are just getting thick—well, one of the reasons is being attached to the damn f@#!*ing flour!

Let me hold you by the hand and walk you through *your* kitchen cleanup. If you live alone or with a roommate or significant other who is joining you on my program, good for you both! Get a big trash bag and start dumping! If you have to consider a partner who won't be participating (or like Susanna, you've got a spouse and kids), enlist their support—and at the very least, plan on rearranging the pantry so you have your own shelf of "safe" foods, while "Danger! High Voltage!" foods get moved to a less accessible area (it's not ideal, but it can work).

I want to warn you, though, this lifestyle can be catching. One client's live-in boyfriend, who originally thought my program extreme ("No pasta," he groaned), soon found himself double-checking the labels of many of the foods he normally enjoyed. People, this happens all the time!—and I love it!

After you start preparing your meals the High Voltage way, chances are it's going to influence your family's way of eating for the better, whether they're ready for it or not!

Managing Your Kitchen Cleanup

What to dump from the pantry: Anything canned—soups, beans, and vegetables (unless they're specifically labeled no salt added). Fruits in heavy syrup. Cranberry sauce. Condiments like ketchup, mustard, and mayonnaise. Breakfast cereal. Waffle, pancake, or cake mixes. Bisquick. Pastas and packaged rice mixes like Rice-A-Roni. Hamburger Helper and other boxed "helper" items. Pasta sauces. Hot cocoa mix. Snack foods like pretzels, potato chips, and corn chips. Prepackaged gravies. Bouillon cubes and broth. Dream Whip and other pudding mixes. Jam, jelly, and regular peanut butter. Pickled vegetables like peppers (unless they're made with no salt). Olives. Bread crumbs. Cracker meal. Flour. Chocolate syrup. Stuffing mixes. Canned fruit filling for pies. Tuna or other canned fish packed in oil. Canned sardines and anchovies.

What to dump from the bread box: Probably everything! Bread, rolls, hamburger and hot dog buns. English muffins, corn muffins, crackers, and flatbreads. Croutons, cookies, cupcakes and other snack cakes. Pies, coffee cake, ladyfingers, cakes (even angel food cake), breadsticks, and salty nacho chips. The only bread crumbs you'll want to keep are the ones you use to feed the birds.

What to dump from the refrigerator: Soy sauce, teriyaki sauce, barbecue sauce, Saucy Susan and steak sauce. Diet and regular sodas. Beer. Cheeses and cheese spreads (except no-salt). Dangerous leftovers like half-eaten lasagna, fried chicken, and two-day-old Chinese food. Yogurt (unless it's the 100-calorie fat-free version). Lunch meats like salami, bologna, and chicken roll. Fruit juice from concentrates (stick to the fresh stuff). Tomato juice and V8 juice. Butter and margarine. Pickles. Whole milk. Salad dressing. Pillsbury's biscuit, dinner roll, and cookie dough (I used to eat that cookie dough raw all the time!). Cool Whip and other whipped toppings.

What to dump from the freezer: All processed foods like frozen vegetables (unless no-salt), frozen pizza and TV dinners. Frozen waffles and pancakes.

Frozen fried chicken and fish sticks. Ice cream. Ice milk. Frozen Milky Ways. Sausage, bacon, and other breakfast meats. Frozen cakes and baked goods. Frozen ravioli. Canned juice. Frozen party hors d'oeuvres. Hot dogs. Frozen french fries and Tater Tots. Ready-made pie crusts. Frozen fruit in syrup (like blueberries or strawberries).

Donate foods to a charity of your choice.
Now some people do protest, "But that's taking away everything that people eat!" Answer: **ABSOLUTELY!** These foods are among the main reasons that we're the fattest nation on the face of the earth and obesity is on the rise! You bet I'm on the warpath to get rid of them. If you tell me that's what everyone eats, I'll tell you it sure is, but look around you and see what eating like that does! I rest my case!

Staying Motivated

In one sense, going on my program is almost like going into therapy. Both involve the process of gaining new skills that allow you to then go off in the world and take better care of yourself. I often tell my clients that I'm a shrink—except that I shrink bodies!

When I work with new clients, as I've mentioned, sometimes they become temporarily dependent on me—which **IS JUST FINE!** While my client is getting rid of old habits and building new ones, we're a team (it's almost as if they're plugging into my strength until they turn theirs on). That can take weeks—or months, depending on the client.

Since I'm not there, at your side, able to keep you **PERSON-ALLY** plugged in, keep this book by your side. Refer to it whenever you need a reminder of why you are doing this and what it can do for you. This is not a book to sit on a shelf. No way! This is your High Voltage handbook, your blueprint for success. Use it! (As I always say, if you don't use it, you'll lose it!) And write to me, c/o my publisher, or e-mail me at HighVoltage@EnergyUp.com. I want to hear from you: I want to hear your stories. I want to help you plug in—that's what an energy conductor does!

Five Days Before Spa Week: Stocking the High Voltage Pantry

After my clients' pantries are emptied, it's important to restock immediately, so that during **SPA WEEK** and thereafter, there is plenty of food to choose from. I don't want clients (or you!) scrambling for the nearest take-out menu at eleven o'clock at night. (Please note: Don't try to restock your pantry at your local 7-Eleven. As of my last visit, the only things they carried that were *somewhat* healthy were some barely acceptable—looking fruit, hard-boiled eggs, and water!)

Often I take my clients shopping to their local supermarket, and to the closest health food store, so we know exactly where to find supplies. One of my clients was living half a block away from a terrific health food store which carried organic produce as well as a wide selection of prepared foods, many of them salt-free. She had never even been inside!—she didn't have a clue! I guess some people have no excuse for the bad food choices they make!

In any case, it's important that *your* pantry and refrigerator be filled to inspire you to cook and eat in a High Voltage way. My program is never about being hungry. The way I see it, some foods and ingredients should always be on hand to jump-start a meal (these are the staples). Other items are the herbs, spices, and seasonings that can make foods more flavorful without adding flour, sugar, salt, and extra fat. The third category is the fresh foods—like fruits, vegetables, dairy products, fish and meats—that you need to replenish frequently. My goal: If you come home late and need to rustle up some dinner, you'll have potatoes on hand to microwave, eggs to scramble, bananas to slice into oatmeal, salad fixings to chop into a big bowl—in short, plenty of choices, all designed to turn a greasy, cheesy quick-delivery pizza into a less appealing option.

The Staples

Rice cakes (plain, not flavored or salted). Puffed rice cereal (unsalted). Salt-free air-popped popcorn (put it in little bags for individual munching). Oatmeal and rolled oats. Water-packed tuna. No-sugar all-fruit jams and jellies and no-salt sugar-free peanut butter. Potatoes and onions. Cornmeal. Brown rice, wild rice, and other grains like quinoa and kasha and couscous. No-salt-added tomato sauce. Black beans, red and white kidney beans, garbanzos, and other beans, no-salt-added only. Water chestnuts. Vegetarian no-salt chili. Carnation powdered skim milk (my mom's favorite—she even puts it in her coffee). And lots and lots of bottled water!

The Flavor Boosters

Balsamic vinegar, rice-wine vinegar, and other flavored vinegars (there are tons!). Unsweetened lime juice. Olive oil, canola oil, no-fat nonstick vegetable oil sprays, sesame oil (not for every day), hot pepper oil. Vanilla extract. Dried spices (I like Mrs. Dash's): cayenne pepper, black pepper, white pepper, garlic powder, onion powder, paprika, coriander, oregano, cinnamon, chili powder, ground cumin, cloves, saffron, thyme, red pepper flakes, mustard powder, and others.

From the Market

Fruits in season like bananas, strawberries, peaches, plums, apples, melons, and oranges (see fruit list in previous chapter, page 107). Lemons and limes for cooking, all year round. Eggs. No-salt, low-fat cottage cheese. No-salt salsa. No-salt hummus. Sweet potatoes. Mushrooms. Eggplant, peppers, broccoli, scallions, carrots, and other veggies (see vegetable list, page 108). No-fat, 100-calorie yogurt. Plain, unflavored yogurt. Low-sodium cheeses (when you can find them). Skinless boneless chicken breasts. Turkey, fresh fish, and shellfish. Lean beef. Fresh horseradish root. Fresh ginger. Fresh herbs like basil, parsley, dill, tarragon, chives, and mint. Skim milk and/or rice milk (I love Rice Dream). No-salt-added, part-skim ricotta cheese. Fresh garlic cloves. Chilies.

Four Days Before Spa Week: Preparing for the Power Surge Workout

Part of **SPA WEEK** involves working out and **FEELING THE ENERGY FLOW!** We've discussed all the details in Chapter Four, but Spa

Week workouts are a jump start to your system and call for something more—more time, more commitment.

To get started, use this day to make a workout plan by figuring out where you're going to do your Spa Week workouts, blocking out the exact times you'll be exercising daily, and getting together any equipment that you may need (clothes, running shoes, small hand weights if you want them, an exercise mat).

When I work out with a client on a full-intensity **SPA WEEK,** we're getting in about three to five hours of exercise per day, often at a health club, a hotel spa, or in a fully equipped exercise room in the client's own home. Nice, right? But what I want you to do is to try to get in half that much—at least an hour and a half, possibly two hours of exercise, beginning on the first day of your **SPA WEEK.**

Volt-Note!

If you haven't been exercising at all, it's a good idea to use the week before Spa Week to gradually add more movement into your life—walking for fifteen minutes to half an hour daily or stretching in the mornings. That way, your Spa Week workout won't be such a shock to your system.

More rules: During Spa Week, at least one hour of your workout should be aerobic (walking or running on a treadmill or around the block, rowing, doing a step routine, using a StairMaster or stationary bike, taking an aerobics class or working out to a video). A must is a sound system or headphones. *Aerobic activity is the only way to burn body fat.* Stretching, toning, and strength-building exercises are terrific—but they don't do the job alone.

Now, you may be wondering how you're going to fit this in—especially if you could never even manage half an hour of exercise, three times a week, before. Well, you're a smart cookie (the only time I use that term), get creative! As I said before, this is not about fitting my program into your established life (which isn't working for you, remember?). **IT'S ABOUT CHANGING YOUR ROUTINE, CHANGING YOUR PATTERNS, CHANGING YOUR LIFE.**

How about waking up an hour earlier and taking a forty-five-minute walk before going to work, fitting in an aerobics class during your lunch hour, and ending the day with an after-hours workout at the local health club? Or taking a brisk walk or bike ride after dinner, instead of vegging out in front of the TV? One of my clients got into the habit of walking on her treadmill during her favorite ten P.M. TV show and eventually worked her time up to the whole hour! Of course, working out to music pushes you harder, but if that was the only time—and she could get in an hour—so be it.

Whatever you decide your routine is going to be, set aside a specific area of your home for your workout.

If you need to buy a step for a step routine, get one.

If you need to pick up an exercise mat and light hand weights, (two, three, five, eight, or ten pounds) and if you want, leg weights (one to five pounds, or even eight pounds if you're extremely strong) from your local sporting goods store, do it.

If walking or running is going to be your aerobic activity of choice, be sure you have headphones and a Walkman, so you can work out to music. Music is the heartbeat of my workout—and of my energy! Besides, if your workout is boring, you probably won't do it. I sometimes think I created my life and my **POWER SURGE** workout so I could listen to music all day!

If you're not working outside the home, or are able to schedule your **SPA WEEK** for a time when you're off from work, your time may be easier to manage.

Check out getting access to a local gym or Y, and plan on spending the mornings there. If you can, do this with a friend who's also going High Voltage! Take a stretch class, take a swim, do aerobics, get an instructor to show you how to use the weight machines—then follow it up with a relaxing whirlpool and steam. Later in the day, plan a bike ride . . . play tennis . . . or dance to rock music in your living room for an hour.

Three Days Before Spa Week: Setting Up a Support System

When you commit to doing **SPA WEEK,** if you live with other people it's up to you to create a supportive environment in your home, which is what I want you to work on today. If you can, get your family, your roommates, your significant other behind you. After all, why shouldn't they support you? It's good for you; and you know, what's good for you could be good for them too.

So use this day to let them know how you feel. Tell your husband how excited you are about the program. Ask your mother not to bring any high-calorie snacks into the house. Remind your boyfriend not to plan on ordering in pizza on Friday night. And, as I mentioned earlier, the ideal scenario is when the people closest to you come on board. I feel best when this happens because I want you to have the best chance of success. A Purdue University study found that dieters with supportive partners lose more weight—thirty percent more!—than those who go it alone (it's especially important if your weight hits a plateau and won't budge!).

If your family or roommates will not be going High Voltage, there are two other scenarios I've encountered.

One is where your family isn't going to undermine you, but they're not going to join you either. If this is not a problem for you, if you can make do with a "safe shelf," and you can prepare non-Voltage meals and snacks for your family and my meals for yourself, that's fine. (I didn't say this was going to be easy, and it's not supposed to be. Nothing really important is! You gotta work hard for everything, but believe me, and believe my other clients—this is worth it: feeling this good about yourself, looking this good, feeling the energy flow is worth it!)

If you don't think you could eat my way while watching your family scarf down burgers or macaroni and cheese, then I suggest you simply explain that this is something you are doing for yourself, and that, for the time being, you are going to be eating your meals in the den or the TV room, or in some other room in your house. One client of mine explained it to her family this way: "This is important to me, and if you respect me, I want you to respect my wishes."

And if they're not willing to support you—even worse, if they're going to undermine your efforts—well, shame on them! What's the big f@#!*ing deal? If they are that selfish and self-centered that they can't help somebody out for one week, well, give me a break! This is one energy blocker that you should be thinking long and hard about!

Two Days Before Spa Week: Recharging Your Environment

But **SPA WEEK** is not just about exercise and eating differently; it's **MORE** than that. It's about changing your eating habits, cleansing your body, getting into the habit of drinking water **(ALL THE TIME, PEO-PLE),** getting into the habit of *moving your body every day*—but it's really about *transformation*. **SPA WEEK** is about caring for yourself, getting you thinking in new ways, getting you *on the track* to a **HIGH VOLTAGE** life. And that is what you're going to be preparing for today.

During Spa Week, you're going to have to clear the decks. You are going to have to make the decision to set aside special time for yourself—**FOR THIS ONE WEEK**—to do things that you don't normally take the time to do. This is important! It is not secondary to the eating and exercise plan . . . **IT IS ALL PART OF THE PLAN TO GET YOU INTO THE NEW HIGH VOLTAGE LIFE THAT YOU ARE CREATING FOR YOURSELF.**

Part of the process involves setting up your home for this special week. I've always believed that environment has a lot to do with keeping your energy level high, which is why I've filled my home with trees and flowers. When I come home, I just breathe in the serenity and beauty of nature all around me—and I feel a sense of tranquillity (not an easy task, since I am based in New York City!). I always think it must be a lot easier to achieve inner tranquillity when you live in the mountains and wake up to gaze out over a breathtaking mountain view, or in a lush tropical setting. But I also believe you can make the most of what you have.

If, like me, your environment doesn't naturally inspire you with a sense of calm, you may have to work to create that mood in your home—with flowers, with light, with candles, and especially with scents. I'm very affected by fragrance and I like to change the scents in my home, depending on the seasons (remember, I don't like gyms because they smell funny). Scent can be a small step—but it's also a powerful one. It gives all my senses a little inner lift to walk into my living room and take in the garden scents of lilacs or roses; to spread a quilt over my bed and get a quick burst of citrus or vanilla sachet; to turn into the hallway and catch the lingering odors of pear or clove or gardenias coming from a scented candle or a bowl of pot-pourri.

Your assignment for today: Think about how to make your environment more nourishing for you. Go shopping and stock up now on scented candles and sachets; look for potpourri rings to place on your lamps and light fixtures (the heat of the light bulb helps diffuse the scent throughout the rooms). Get ready to set out vases of fresh flowers—in the bedroom, in the bathroom (these can be positive signals, reminders that you are doing something special for yourself this week). You might even arrange with your local florist to have fresh flowers delivered to your home on day three—a midweek reward for yourself for sticking to **SPA WEEK**—and moving ahead! Plants and flowers are living things—they'll respond to your energy too. Do I talk to my plants? You betcha!

One Day Before Spa Week: Planning Your Beauty Regimen

Client **SPA WEEKS** are long on activity, but they're also **VERY** long on luxury! Massages every day (for me *and* my client—after all, everything they do, I do). Facials. Body wraps. All sorts of feel-good treatments that create pleasure and promote body awareness. So for those of you doing your **SPA WEEK** at home, I want you to plan on giving yourself at least one "spa" beauty treatment per day.

Where, you may be wondering again, is all this time coming from? That's what you're going to be figuring out today. Part of **SPA WEEK** is learning to use your down time to refresh and renew yourself, rather than just melting down in front of the TV and feeding yourself (which is what most people do in their down time!). But once again, we're changing established patterns here. Aren't you tired of being tired? Your old ways just don't cut it!

So just as you blocked out time on your calendar when you're going to be doing your daily workouts, I want you to schedule in a daily beauty treatment. Make that time a gift to yourself! For example, on the first day of Spa Week, how about locking the door, turning off the phone, putting the kids to bed, twisting your hair up in a favorite scarf, lighting a scented candle, and indulging yourself in a fragrant bath, filled with aromatic bath salts and bubbles. I want you to plan something special for each and every day—then, make a list and stock up on any special supplies or materials you're going to need (like candles, bath salts or bubbles, a new facial masque, a loofah, aromatic herbs, scented oils, and the like). If you're able to, now is the time to make any special appointments you've decided to enjoy on your Spa Week, like a massage, manicure, or pedicure, or even a full "day of beauty" at your local day spa or salon. The point is to prepare ahead and make it part of your Spa Week plan.

What sorts of things work? Paint your toenails. Try aromatherapy. Read a magazine. Work on your affirmations. Plan your next day. In short, get involved in caring for yourself as opposed to doing something destructive—like munching crackers, cupcakes, or chips, or gossiping on the phone. **REMEMBER THAT THE MOST IMPORTANT RELATIONSHIP YOU EVER HAVE ON THIS PLANET IS THE ONE YOU HAVE WITH YOURSELF!**

At-Home Beauty Treatments for SPA WEEK

Here are some typical Spa Week beauty activities that I've worked out for you, based on what I do with my clients. Use my list as a model to create one that works for you.

1. Treat yourself to a skin-nourishing, deep-cleansing facial masque. Smooth it on; give it lots of time to dry while you amuse yourself by painting your toenails in a color you've never tried before. Rinse the masque off; pat your face dry. If you don't care to buy a commercial masque, how about whipping one up yourself with natural ingredients from your kitchen, like oatmeal, egg whites, or papaya? Here's one I've liked for years. For dry skin, take warm, fresh applesauce and mix it with wheat germ to make a paste; apply it to your skin. Let it set till dry; rinse (to soothe sunburned skin, substitute oatmeal for wheat germ). For oily skin, peel and remove the seeds from a large tomato; mash the firm tomato pulp with enough oatmeal to make a thick but smooth paste. Smooth it on your skin; let it dry; rinse with warm water.

2. Loofah your body in the shower tonight; gently rub your elbows and knees with pumice till you are as smooth as silk. Afterwards, apply a feel-good body masque; follow up with a creamy, scented body lotion (apply in long strokes while your skin is still damp to get the most moisturizing benefits).

3. Steam yourself clean. When I'm with a client at a hotel spa or health club, we have the luxury of popping in and out of steam rooms (and Jacuzzis) all day, so our skin gets the wonderful, cleansing benefits of all that steam. Here's an at-home facial steam that works: Place a big pot of water on the stove; heat it to a boil; remove the pot from the heat, place a towel over your head, and lean over the pot, keeping your face about six inches from the water. Steam for five minutes; close your pores with a splash of cold water. Better yet, throw some yummy herbs like lavender, chamomile, or rosemary into the water.

4. Spruce up your fingers and toes with a professional manicure and pedicure. If you can, have someone come to your home and do it for you. After all, this is **SPA WEEK**; this is how you're rewarding yourself—not with cake or food, but with something that is GOOD for your body. Follow up with a lavender oil-and-bubble bath (candles, music, a tall glass of sparkling water with a slice of orange and a strawberry) to make you feel wonderful. Close the door. Don't hurry. Relaxxxx . . .

5. Give your hair a special hot oil treatment or deep conditioning—the kind you only do once every three months or so (wrap your head in cellophane to encourage penetration). While the hair conditioner is working, give yourself a foot massage (use your favorite scented lotion) or, if money is not an issue, have a practitioner come to your home for a reflexology (foot massage) treatment.

6. If you can afford it, have a massage. Swedish, deep-tissue, shiatsu, reiki—there's a whole fabulous world of massage techniques to explore. Plus, massage is not a frivolous indulgence: it releases tension and stress, soothes workout-tired muscles, *and* is a divine way of rewarding yourself. If you've never had a massage before, it's worth saving up for. And today, many massage professionals will come to your home—not for what you think! (I'm sure massage parlor pros are available for *that* too, but that's not what we're talking about here!) If a massage is just not in the financial stars for you right now, buy a how-to massage book and rope a special friend into giving you one (you'll promise, of course, to return the favor).

7. To experience all of the above, make an appointment for a complete "day of beauty" at any of the excellent day spas that are cropping up in cities all over the country (I can't think of a better time than Spa Week to put something like this on your schedule). One of my favorites is Georgette Klinger's, which has outposts across the country, and is now run by her daughter Katherine, who, in addition to being beautiful, happens to be a real sweetheart. The last time I was in Beverly Hills, we had lunch together and she gave me a day of beauty to try at the New York salon. I heartily recommend it!

8. Expand your mind. **SPA WEEK** is a week of discovery on all levels. Physical fitness conditions the body, but spiritual fitness nourishes the soul! In addition to adding at least an hour and a half to two hours of exercise activity to your life, try to engage in an activity that promotes spiritual awareness and relaxation at least once during the week, like yoga, tai chi, or meditation. Or try something offbeat . . . New Age . . . a little unusual perhaps . . . but that's also kind of fun. Spirit dancing, for example, is a unique, healing dance class (and high-energy workout!) that combines free-flowing yoga, dance, and low-impact aerobics in a way that allows you to reconnect with your body and reclaim your soul (not unlike my nightclub energy concerts!). Or have your palm read—or your tea leaves. Your handwriting analyzed. Your astrological chart done (I'm a dollar sign!). Look into tarot cards, the *I Ching,* ancient runes, or even get a referral to a psychic.

   Even if you don't believe in any of these things, exploration can be fun. And you never know, sometimes something just clicks. Besides, my name is **HIGH VOLTAGE**—as I said earlier, I'm a born-again something—I just don't know what. (If you've never done any of the above before, ask your friends about it. You just may be surprised at who is into this, but was too embarrassed to ever let on).

It's Spa Week!

It's here—Spa Week—your intense immersion into my program. If you've done your homework on your countdown to Spa Week, you should be well stocked up with water, ready with your workout and beauty schedule, and rarin' to go. During Spa Week, you're going to:

- Say your affirmations, at least twice a day (in the morning when you wake up, before you go to bed at night, as needed during the day).
- Eat according to my Star Power Plan (see sample menu on pages 196–98) but with special only-on-Spa-Week guidelines. Reread those Ten Commandments, page 117, and keep them handy in your purse when you go out).
- Work out for one and a half to two hours a day (part aerobic, part Power Surge). Go back to Chapter Six, page 134, and review the Power Surge exercises.
- Indulge in one beauty treatment per day.
- Keep working on those energy blocks. Set aside some time to think about and work on them every day.
- Drink water, water, water. This is the week when you're going to make it a habit for life!

**Spa Week
Daily Checklist**

Affirmations (twice a day)
Star Power Eating (see Seven-Day Jump-start Menu, page 196)
Power Surge Workout, page 134, (one and a half to two hours a day)
Beauty Treatment (once a day)
Water (six to eight eight-ounce bottles a day)

Eating During SPA WEEK

On **SPA WEEK,** my chefs specialize in meals at their most elegant, colorful, and flavorful. Everything must be beautifully prepared (the presentation is part of the treat), so that the food satisfies the eyes as well as the mouth. While my clients are not going to be thinking about food all day—when it *is* time to eat, I want them to be delighted by the colors, the fragrance, the look of the food, as well as the taste.

On **SPA WEEK,** we go all out: My chef prepares fabulous entrees, soups, different hors d'oeuvres with great dips using every kind of herb on the planet, crisp, thin-as-the-air vegetable chips, and sumptuous salsas. The presentation is magnificent! Everything is just a little fresher, more imaginatively prepared, more colorful than usual—you feel like you're in a four-star restaurant (if I didn't tell people that this food was healthy, wonderful, and good for you, they would never know!).

But everything has to be appealing. The clients who hire me, after all, are accustomed to being served at top restaurants like Le Cirque, La Grenouille, and "21"!

Again, I'm aiming to please *all* the senses. We dine with candles—*always*. And with flowers on the table. The ingredients are always fresh and the menu relies heavily on fish, shellfish, fruits and vegetables (organic when possible), and light, elegant desserts. (This is not about being hungry—in fact, many of my clients are concerned that there is too much food!). We also serve our main meal at midday rather than in the evening, an old-time custom that I'd like to see revived. That way, we refuel our bodies—and use our fuel during the day, instead of just going to sleep after a big meal. We also use luncheon plates, to make us feel our plates are full, rather than full-sized dinner plates. It's a psychological thing—and one well worth getting used to.

Over the years, the chefs I work with have created many wonderful **SPA** menus. Below is a typical seven-day menu, each day averaging under 1000 calories, with recipes created to specifications by Victor Swainson, one of my most talented, creative (not to mention gorgeous!) chefs. My clients love him! Each of the dishes follows my Star, is naturally low in fat, and of course, keeps in mind my three no-no's. But each is so flavorful that I promise you won't ever know the difference! Follow this menu or adapt it to your own tastes, or use it as a springboard to help create your own High Voltage meals (plus, you'll find boldface recipes which appear in the Recipes on page 236).

Along with the **SPA WEEK** menu, be sure to drink your six to eight glasses of water a day. I want you to carry that water bottle with you everywhere—to the bathroom, to the living room, to the office. Put a bottle on your bedside table, near the chair where you read the evening paper, in the TV room, and in the area where you plan to do your workout. **THIS** is a biggie, people, I can't emphasize it enough. My program will **NOT WORK** without water. (I was stunned one time when a client showed up with a Chanel water carrier—with a $1,400 price tag. This is certainly not required!)

Not on Spa Week

Throughout these pages, I've referred to certain foods that I (reluctantly) allow on my High Voltage maintenance program when your weight is where you want it to be, but not on **SPA WEEK,** which is your week of purification and transformation. Below is a listing of those "never on Spa Week" items, in addition to my no flour, and no added sugar or salt guidelines.

- No soba, rice-flour, or buckwheat noodles or other items made from alternatives to wheat flour.
- No flour-free muffins or anything that resembles conventional baked goods.
- No white rice (brown rice only, please).
- No sugar substitutes like Sweet'n Low or Equal.
- No alcohol whatsoever (you know how I feel about this!).
- No salt substitutes.
- No nuts or nut butters (even if they're salt-free).
- No mustard, Worcestershire sauce, or other low-salt condiments.
- No low-sodium cheese (only salt-free cheeses, please).
- No beef, lamb, pork, goose, or duck.

Key for Recipes:

Boldface means the recipe for this dish can be found in the Recipes section on the page indicated.

Seven-Day Jump-start Menu

Day 1

¾ cup rolled oat cereal with ½ cup skim milk (sprinkle with cinnamon, vanilla extract, ¼ cup chopped apples and raisins, 1 teaspoon shredded coconut)

Fresh citrus salad

Coffee or Tea

Green salad with spicy popcorn "croutons"

Pan-Roasted Monkfish with Wild Mushroom Ragout (p. 236)

Baked Red and Yellow Tomatoes (p. 237)

Couscous-stuffed artichokes

Frisée lettuce with **Lemon-Basil Vinaigrette** (p. 237)

Whipped Strawberry "Mousse" (p. 238)

Day 2

High Voltage Spa "Morning Sunrise" shake (½ cup almond milk, ½ cup strawberries with ice cubes in blender)

Coffee or tea

Scallion-Shrimp Pancakes (p. 238)
Sautéed Zucchini (p. 239)
Romaine lettuce and Vidalia onion with **Lemon-Basil Vinaigrette** (p. 237)

Curried Carrot and Acorn Squash Soup (p. 239)
6-Vegetable Terrine with Peppered Fresh Tomato Sauce (p. 240)
Peach sorbet with white grape juice sweetener

Day 3
Grapefruit juice
½ cup multigrain oatmeal with sliced peaches
Coffee or tea

Grilled Tuna with Chickpeas and Spinach (p. 241)
Roast beets with haricots verts, with **Shallot-Mustard Vinaigrette** (p. 242)

Refreshing Chilled Cucumber-Basil Soup (p. 242)
Spinach salad with **Garlic Herb Dressing** (p. 243)
Brown Rice with Lemon-Pepper Relish (p. 243)
Iced yogurt parfait with berries

Day 4
Millet porridge (almond milk, cinnamon, and vanilla, and chopped dates)
Sliced papaya, mango, and banana "cocktail"
Coffee or tea

Spaghetti squash with **Tomato Sauce with Mushrooms** (p. 244)
Baby greens with plum tomatoes and **Roasted Red Pepper Vinaigrette** (p. 245)

Delicious Tuscan Bean Soup (p. 245)
Italian Vegetable Frittata (p. 246)
Frozen strawberries mixed with orange wedges

Day 5
Crunchy apple-pear-berry yogurt parfait (sliced apples, pears, blueberries, and raspberries, swirled with unflavored yogurt and a teaspoon of wheat germ)
Coffee or tea

Grilled chicken breast with seasonal herbs topped with **Peach Salsa** (p. 246)
Lightly steamed peas
Curried Banana (p. 247)

Peppery Corn Chowder (p. 247)
Green salad with **Red Onion Dressing** (p. 248)
Mixed Berries with Scarlet Strawberry Sauce (p. 248)

Day 6
Sliced hard-boiled egg
Grapefruit and orange sections
Coffee or tea

Voltage Chicken with Vegetables and Couscous (p. 249)
Steamed spinach with garlic and lemon
Crunchy Raw Vegetable Slaw (p. 250)

197

Cold Asparagus Soup (p. 250)
Energy Antipasto Dinner (p. 251)
Cappuccino pudding (see Fifty-one Food Tips,
    p. 214)

Day 7
Mushroom egg-white omelet
½ cup mixed blackberries, raspberries, and kiwi
    slices
Coffee or tea

Salmon Steak with Citrus Vinaigrette (p. 252)
St. Tropez Vegetables (p. 252)
Tricolor salad

Poached Scallops with Green Sauce (p. 253)
Emerald Rice (p. 253)
Chilled yogurt (swirl with sugar-free raspberry
    jam, sprinkle with toasted wheat germ)

Reality Check

When clients first make the decision to go on my program, if they're not going away to a spa, I suggest avoiding social events for the first few days (if they can't get away, and are really trying to make this fundamental change in their behavior, it's important to stay away from as many outside energy influences as possible).

The same thing applies to you. Understand, what you're doing is like starting a journey. It's a transformation. I always say to my clients that I am not putting them on a diet, I am showing them a different way to live!

To get the total benefits of **SPA WEEK,** it's ideal if you can take the week off, so your focus is on yourself—not on your job, not on your school, family, or work obligations. But—reality!—life is not always ideal! If that's just not possible, consider the following strategies for adapting **SPA WEEK** activities to real life.

If your job, school, or family makes it totally impossible to get in the one and a half to two hours of exercise per day that **SPA WEEK** calls for, plus one hour of beauty, I understand. Instead, try for an exercise *hour*—a half hour in the morning, a half hour sometime during the rest of the day.

Don't neglect the pampering, though. Give yourself your beauty treatment before you go to bed (you deserve it!).

As for the menu, during client **SPA WEEKS,** our main meal is at midday. This may be impossible for you if you work in an office and are brown-bagging it. If that's the case, during your **SPA WEEK,** have your **SPA** breakfast, make a simplified lunch that you can bring with you and put in the office refrigerator or reheat in the office microwave, and prepare our luxurious **SPA** lunch as your dinner, once you get home. Below are five in-the-office **SPA** lunch suggestions:

1. 100-calorie yogurt, a green salad, and an orange.
2. Baked potato topped with a can of water-packed tuna and a dollop of homemade salsa, a banana for dessert.
3. Grilled chicken breast, ½ cup brown rice, green salad with balsamic dressing, and a clementine.
4. Half a cantaloupe stuffed with berries, plus ½ cup low-fat, no-salt cottage cheese.
5. Spinach-and-tomato salad with sliced hard-boiled egg, rice cake with hummus, peach or plum.

And drink bottled or filtered water all the time!

Take Credit for All You've Accomplished

At the end of **SPA WEEK,** the conversations I have with clients are totally different from the ones we had when we began because I'm talking to a different person—with a different outlook

> **Volt-Note!**
>
> Facing the scale: Some fitness regimes say, "Stay away from the scale." I don't believe in that. When we start **SPA WEEK,** unless clients are totally scale-phobic (yes, some people are!), I ask that they write down their starting weight, and weigh themselves once a day, same time, **EVERY** morning thereafter. Some people may be uncomfortable with this at first (they just don't want to know). But I insist, because I know their weight is going to come down immediately as we eliminate the salt and the flour. (Yes, I know it's just water weight at first, but the psychological impact of that early loss can be a big motivating factor.) Plus, if you keep with the program, keep eating my way after **SPA WEEK,** it's not going to come back.
>
> Of course, over the years, I have dealt with clients who were truly compulsive about the numbers on the scale. I had one client who kept three scales in her home (yes, it is possible to get a little neurotic about this!). The half-pound or pound difference among them soon drove her crazy. At one point, she was sending drivers all over town to pick up the most expensive scales they could find in order to get an accurate reading (sometimes the more money you have, the crazier you get). But I called a stop to that, pronto. "We'll use just one scale and that's it," I told her. "And we're not going to obsess about half a pound up or half a pound down. It just doesn't matter!"

forming. I have to tell you, to see this happening is always exciting to me. After the end of the week (or two), I see a gleam in their eyes; they're losing their compulsions about food because they **NOW KNOW THEY CAN DO THIS!** In the beginning, it's always, "Oh, I'll never be able to keep this up." But by the fourth day, it's like, "Oh God, I feel so much better. This isn't so difficult!" And by the end, I hear, "I just don't want to eat that way anymore!" (with flour, sugar, and salt they mean).

So go with the flow: **LET IT HAPPEN TO YOU TOO.** You're going to like the way you feel so much that you're not going to want to turn back. By the end of the week, I want you to start equating cake with lack of energy. Potato chips with feeling sick. We're changing the tapes in your brain!

Remember, if you don't think you could do this program forever, well, you're gonna do it one day at a time. Any recovery program is built on that premise.

I always tell people that many of the issues they have now ("I hate rice cakes, I can't eat these!" or "I can't go without flour!") are going to disappear. In the beginning, sure, all of my ideas seem foreign to conventional ways of thinking. But after a few days, it won't feel foreign anymore. There are plenty of other foods to eat. There are plenty of other things to do. Women notice their cellulite starting to go down; men notice their middles aren't so thick anymore. All of a sudden you'll be looking at bread . . . at salt . . . and at sugar differently (as your enemy)!

So that's the process. And it works; it *will* get you results. If it didn't, my clients would tell me to f@#!* off. And you would too.

After Spa Week: Keep Listening to Your Body

SPA WEEK is your intense transformation week—the activity level is high (one and a half to two hours per day, and three to five hours for clients!); the daily calorie count is low (around 800 to 1000 calories per day). **Its purpose is to help you stop and listen to your body**—cleanse your system, break old habits, begin new ones—and open your mind to accepting a whole new way of life.

After **SPA WEEK,** you should be feeling energized. Lighter. Thinner. And motivated! As you move into incorporating these principles into real life, here's what you need to do.

- You need to keep up your affirmations. That's a BIG source of your inner energy!
- I want you to try to stay with at least 30 minutes of aerobic exercise daily—and plenty of stretching (but more than 30 minutes is always better, people!).
- And you need to follow my Ten Commandments, keeping your pantry stocked in a High Voltage way, cooking in a way that boosts flavor, loses fat, and keeps your energy up! It's your fuel—let's make it the best fuel it can be. Personally, I choose to think of myself as a sleek Ferrari, not a rusted-up dump truck!

So turn to the next chapter and let's talk about how to keep your new High Voltage ways going.

ENERGY UP! WHOO!

Chapter 8

MAINTAINING A **HIGH** VOLTAGE **LIFE**STYLE

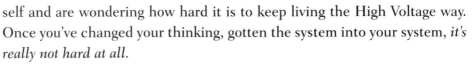

After you have made it through **SPA WEEK,** you are probably feeling pretty good about yourself and are wondering how hard it is to keep living the High Voltage way. Once you've changed your thinking, gotten the system into your system, *it's really not hard at all.*

The Star Power Plan is just a new way of doing things—and like all new things, it may seem difficult at first. That's why, in this chapter, in addition to my Fifty-one Food Tips to get you started, you'll find recipes for tasty meals to prepare the High Voltage way. I'm quite aware that I spend a lot of time telling people what **NOT** to do—well, here's how to make it all work on a daily basis. . . .

The fact is, once you eliminate processed "convenience" foods, most of the food you regularly enjoy, like chicken, fish, meat, vegetables, rice, and other grains, **ARE FINE ALL BY THEMSELVES.** The problems come into play in terms of how you cook them, what you cook them with, or especially, what you spoon over them afterwards.

Don't Eliminate Any Food Group

On the Star Power Plan, I don't eliminate any single food group or category. I'm always suspicious (you should be too) of any so-called diet that advises you to cut out an entire food category or categories—like no more carbohydrates, ever! Ridiculous! Or eat only fruit. Or only vegetables. Even though I say no sugar and no salt (*nonnegotiable!*), it's no *added* sugar and salt. You get plenty of natural sugars from fruits, and natural sodium in vegetables, eggs, and other foods. You get starches—not from bread or pasta, but from rice and grains, potatoes and yams (all loaded with nutrients straight from the good earth!). I've even bent so far as to allow rice cakes—in moderation, of course. I'd love you to go for the brown-rice cakes, but frankly, I'm not going to battle with you over a rice cake—as long as they're salt-and-sugar-free. No more than three a day, please.

The Star Power Plan includes chicken, beef, fish, and even eggs. I like to substitute egg whites in recipes that call for whole eggs (if you're watching cholesterol, limit your eggs to no more than two a week). Some people even find that cholesterol is not much of an issue for them, once they start eating in a naturally healthy, naturally low-in-fat way.

Finally, the Star Power Plan includes dairy products for calcium, and even fats (remember, we need fats in our diet for healthy skin, hair, nails—and for your organs to function, guys!). We just don't need as much fat as most people are eating, like all those fatty cheeses.

If you have a weakness for cheese, by the way, while it's not a big part of my program, it's not eliminated either. Just skip the salty ones, and seek out no-salt or low-salt, low-fat versions (more and more of which are coming on the market all the time).

So, what's missing? Flour, sugar, and salt. *That's it*. If you start eating the High Voltage way, your diet will be naturally low in calories and fat and give you plenty of fiber (you're getting it in vegetables, fruits, and grains) and enough protein (don't need all that much!), along with fats and calcium (in low-fat cheese, nonfat yogurt, and skim milk, powdered or fresh—one of the few things that come in a box I don't go to battle over).

Maintaining

Until your weight is where you want it to be, stick with Star Power, drink water (it really works!), and use your common sense as to slight variations here and there (like I said before, unless you're in a totally controlled environment—like on a **SPA WEEK** with me and my chef!—salt is a toughie!).

But be forewarned: A cup of commercial cereal for breakfast, for example, may not seem like much, but it's a **BIG MISTAKE.** It's going to start you off wrong from the get-go, drag you down—mind, body and spirit—**BIG-TIME.** Get your body and your brain where you want them to be—and the energy to stick with Star Power and follow the Ten Commandments will soon start generating.

Once your energy is up—and your weight down—stay with the Star Power Plan, but add a little more protein, or a larger portion of grain. After three or four months—depending on how much weight you want to lose, of course—you should be able to determine what your body can handle. If your weight goes up more than two or three pounds (for women, I'm not talking about the normal fluctuations that come with your menstrual cycle, or other natural variations), go back to the original Star Power Plan. *It really is your guiding star.*

Forget Plain Jane Food, Get Creative

Does the food have to be plain? No f@#!*ing way! In fact, it should taste better and more flavorful than the taste bud–deadening foods most people are used to (your food's not really tasty, guys, it's just salty!).

My chefs serve up spicy curries, delicious roasted garlic (which I love eating just plain!), fiery southwestern and even Cajun-style specialties. I have worked with so many creative chefs over the years, who have accompanied me on **SPA WEEKS,** that I have collected quite a notebook of recipes and food tips. Many of my clients have gotten quite creative too, all within Star Power guidelines.

For dessert, how about a simple apple-ginger compote: coarsely chopped apples, tossed with a little natural apple or white grape juice and sprinkled with cinnamon and fresh ginger?

Or chop some fresh dill in with boiled new potatoes, sliced cucumbers, chopped red and yellow peppers, and vinegar, for a healthy potato salad.

Throw a handful of spicy popcorn on a green salad to take the place of fried croutons. My favorite air-popped popcorn is called Nude Food from Robert's American Gourmet. I buy the superspicy Fra Diavolo version, which gets its fire from paprika and red pepper. The whole big bag (it only weights two ounces, but it's the same size as an eight-ounce bag of pretzels or chips, guys!—popcorn is light but bulky stuff) has only 200 calories and just a pinch of canola oil. You can even eat the whole bag at a single sitting— and sometimes I do! (If you have trouble drinking all your water, this popcorn is so spicy it will have you downing gallons in no time!) This is what I smuggle into my local movie theater.

Just be prepared—especially in the first three months, don't leave the day's meal plans to chance. Without getting obsessed about it, until High Voltage eating comes naturally (and even afterwards, when it does), it's perfectly natural to plan the food you're going to eat. After all, you plan what you're going to wear, the people you're going to see each week, your work schedule, the movies or activities in which you're going to participate—*why not your food?*

Thinking through meals in advance can help you cope with high-risk meals like business lunches, holiday dinners, or other special occasions. If you know you're going to be someplace that offers minimal choice when it comes to High Voltage food (like in a shopping mall), tuck some fruit, a hard-boiled egg, rice cakes, cut-up veggies, or a yogurt into your bag. Bring your water and your own no-salt popcorn to the movies.

Don't get trapped when you're traveling either. My clients call ahead to the airlines and order a special meal—salt-free or vegetarian or a fresh fruit plate. It's really **NOT A BIG DEAL.** Just be sure to bring along plenty of fresh fruit anyway—airline food, special meals or not, while not **DANGER! HIGH VOLTAGE!** still basically sucks.

Finally, I am well aware that my way of eating is different from the way you've been brought up, even from the so-called healthy-eating diets of the last decade. Thank God! But once again, look around you: by eating that way, people's bodies have gotten bigger, not better! It's time to try a new way to get this country moving, to get our energies flowing, to get our **ENERGY UP!**

As far as I'm concerned, we've been on brownout . . . and we're moving dangerously close to a blackout anytime now! I try to make this all as much fun as possible—you've got Star Power, Spa Week, the High Voltage Ten Commandments, Danger! High Voltage! reminders, food that's dead or alive—and of course, my "Whoo!"—but believe me, this issue is as serious as a heart attack. I mean it. Again, as I said before, remember my company name—**DFWM!** Whoo!

Reality Check: Life's Little Inconsistencies

Know the old saying—that consistency is the hobgoblin of petty minds? Well, even if you don't, for the most part, I think you'll find the **STAR** Plan *damn* consistent. It's quick, it's easy, the choices are made for you, all you have to remember (or forget about!) are those three white powders (Danger! High Voltage!).

And once you've gotten it down, **YOU CAN SPEND YOUR TIME THINKING ABOUT MORE IMPORTANT THINGS IN YOUR LIFE THAN JUST FOOD.**

Still, here's a **REALITY CHECK**—to help bring Star Power within your reach. It will help to explain some of the little inconsistencies that make life interesting.

1. *Rice cakes:* Yes, I know that just like bagels, they fall into the carbohydrate category—one of those starches that, like sugar, enter the bloodstream fast, convert to sugar, then to fat in a flash. That's why I don't want you eating more than three a day. Ideal world: Look for brown- or wild-rice cakes. Reality: As I said before, I'm not going to go to war with you over a white-rice cake! If you can't stick with three a day, don't eat them!

2. *Baked potatoes:* Same thing as above. Yes, it's one of those carbs. But we live in the real world, people. And the fact that potatoes are natural goes a long way with me.

3. *Sushi:* Was I upset when I found my fingers were puffy with water weight the day after my little sushi lunch! Later, I found out it wasn't the sushi, but all that salty pickled ginger that goes along with it. The white rice in the sushi—puh-leeze. I'm not going to battle over that one either. I've got more important fish to fry. (Of course, I wouldn't be frying my fish, but you know what I mean.)

4. *Coffee and tea:* Once again, in that perfect world, coffee and tea wouldn't be issues (yes, they are drugs!). But, people, not even High Voltage is perfect!—not yet, anyway. I do drink coffee and unless it disagrees with you, I'm not going to take it away. Same goes for tea, although if you haven't as yet, I wish you'd explore the world of delicious flavors of herbal teas. Watch out for commercial, bottled iced tea drinks, though. One of my new clients was very happy filling up on her favorite flavored bottled tea—until she read the label, saw the sugar, and saw the light!

5. *Tuna in a can:* Yes, it's a canned food. Technically dead. But in the real world, in a pinch, it's handy to have a few cans of these in your cupboard. I always do! Just be sure to buy it packed in water (not oil!) and then rinse it and pat it with a paper towel to get as much of the salt off as you can. This has saved my ass many times, when I had nothing else in the house to eat or when I was traveling and had to grab something from a deli on the run.

6. *Mustard:* I've stayed away from mustard because I am so supersensitive to salt, but to be honest, mustard is considered one of the "better" condiments because it's high on flavor, doesn't have much fat, and can be low in sodium (averaging from 50 to 130mg per teaspoon)—*if and only if you use just a teaspoon.* So use it to pep up a salad dressing or a

marinade, but don't slather it on everything (not that there's anything to slather it on—no sandwiches, remember!). And—need I say it?—never on **SPA WEEK,** or whenever you're trying to drop a few pounds fast. This applies, by the way to Worcestershire sauce—a terrific flavor enhancer when you're cooking. Lea & Perrins Worcestershire has 5 calories per teaspoon, no fat, 1 lonely gram of sugar and 65mg of sodium. Just don't abuse the privilege! Which brings me to . . .

7. *Tortilla chips:* The baked-without-salt ones, of course. Technically, they're safe (gotta hand it to the companies that are making them). But these are one of those easy-to-abuse foods, along with no-salt, oil-free potato chips, veggie chips, and similar snacks. If you're a food addict, watch your step here. Don't scarf down a bag—or two—and say that High Voltage says it's okay. It's not. They **STILL HAVE CALORIES!** I seldom buy them anymore myself, because believe it or not, I can't control myself (as you know, I'm low on self-control!).

8. *Artificial sweeteners:* I stand by what I said before. In a perfect world, no. On **SPA WEEK,** no. In reality: If you gotta, you gotta. But I don't want to hear about it.

9. *Rice milk:* Yes, yes, yes, I know it has sea salt added. This is a case where I care more about avoiding the hormones and chemicals in milk than about a pinch of sea salt (common sense, remember!). Besides, the taste is so luscious and sweet (especially the vanilla!) . . . and since I do work out more than the average person, this has become one of my personal treats. Inconsistent, perhaps, but this is not an exact science.

Fifty-one High Voltage Food Tips

These are some of the food tricks I've compiled over the years—some are from my own little bag of tricks; some are from my mother's bag of tricks; others have been developed by my spa chefs; still others I've learned at spas at which I've been a guest; and still others have been given to me by creative clients who have taken my Star to new heights. I'm always thrilled when a client sends me a new recipe or tip made according to Spa Power guidelines. It's a real turn-on! (I hope to hear from you too.)

Since not all my clients have chefs (although many do!), and many are too busy to cook or are just not that accomplished in the kitchen, I've sometimes looked for healthy-food home-delivery services, which are cropping up all over the country. These services actually deliver heart-healthy, body-healthy, portion-controlled meals by the week or by the month. One that I've recommended to my New York clients that has proven to be a winner is HeartSmart, based in Southampton, Long Island. Chef/owner Jim Jondreau specializes in delicious, low-fat dishes; I was so impressed that I asked him to revise some of them to conform with my Star Power Plan. You'll find them interspersed in our Thirty-Day Menu, with easy-to-follow recipes included in our Recipes. If this sort of service is of interest to you—start looking around. Ask at your local health food store, or check in the back of local papers under food services.

As for organic foods: I always recommend them and I hope you'll look for them in your local supermarket or farmers' market. If you can't find them, pick up a copy of *Green Groceries: A Mail Order Guide to Organic Foods,* by Jeanne Heifetz, which lists hundreds of sources.

Fifty-one Tips

1. Instead of conventional french fries—too much oil, and the wrong kind, plus salt!—try making them this way: Cut potatoes into slices or strips; boil them till they are cooked halfway, and remove from pot. Place on a baking pan, season to taste with a teaspoon of peanut oil, cayenne pepper, and a little Mrs. Dash (that's the salt-free seasoning I use), and bake at 350–375 degrees till crispy and golden.

2. My chefs also make great vegetable chips: Boil sweet potatoes, celery root, beets, plantain, and carrots separately till cooked but not mushy (they have to be firm); then slice and toss with oil and spices (see above) and bake *slowly* at 275 degrees till light brown (watch these—if you burn them, the taste will be bitter).

3. When you're boiling potatoes, put a whole onion and a bay leaf in the pot, and boil together. Use the stock as a base for a healthy, salt-free vegetable soup.

4. To add a healthy zing to foods, try fresh grated horseradish root (if you use prepared horseradish, squeeze and rinse first to remove as much salt as possible). Use it as a crust for fish or chicken (mix with cornmeal, tarragon parsley, cayenne, cumin, and water or vinegar into a paste, rub over the surface, and bake. Instead of water or vinegar, you could also try a bit of lemon juice, olive oil, or another flavored oil).

5. Another horseradish tip: Use a teaspoon of horseradish to poach fish, add a little fire to cooked vegetables, or as a flavor replacement for salt. Combine with apple cider vinegar or rice-wine vinegar, add pepper, rosemary, and thyme. Again, this is not about bland; we're really giving food a zap here!

6. Ditto for dill—fresh, not dried. It's nice with fish or shrimp, or stirred into icy cold unflavored yogurt with chopped cucumbers and a splash of lemon juice.

7. To flavor steamed vegetables, forget about salt and butter. Instead, try a twist of lemon zest, a splash of orange juice, a sprinkling of sesame seeds, or a couple of drops of extra-virgin olive oil. Or serve veggies up with a delicious onion coulis: Take 3 large onions; bake till golden, then put in the blender. Add a teaspoon of olive oil, ¼ cup lemon juice, ⅓ cup vinegar, ½ cup water, and a pinch of cayenne pepper, white and black peppers, or jalapeño pepper.

8. A super snack you may not know about: crunchy pea mix made from green peas, adzuki, and lentils. You can find these in the organic section of your regular supermarket. They are so delicious that they really bring home the message that you can eat anything you want—*you'll just want different things!*

9. To me, salsa (chopped peppers, tomatoes, onions, and spices) is like magic— better than ketchup, mustard, and mayonnaise all put together (okay, I do like my food hot and spicy!). But there's something about salsa that really wakes you up. I serve it with egg-white omelets or scrambled eggs, toss it on a side dish

of steamed or sautéed vegetables, and even use it to spice up soup! Look for brands that have no added oil, no sugar, and low sodium (Newman's Own Bandito is one; Enrico's salsa is another).

10. Tofu is a mouthful of protein and it takes on the flavor of whatever you combine it with. This is one of my favorite tricks and it takes just thirty seconds (that's the kind of cook I am). Cut off a chunk of tofu packed in water; cube it up; add 2 tablespoons of your favorite salsa, stir, and voilà! It's a terrific minimeal—one I use often! And would you believe that tofu can replace the taste of ice cream in a blender shake? Well, try it, for a creamy and rich, thick texture.

11. Don't confine your salsa to just the popular tomato kind—there's corn salsa, mango salsa, even berry salsa, all made with lemon juice, vinegar, and spices (serve them with chicken or fish to add just that little flavor boost). To make 2 cups of peach salsa (nice with chicken): Combine 4 medium peaches, pitted and chopped, ⅓ cup green peppers, ⅔ cup chopped red onion, 3 tablespoons lemon juice, 2 tablespoons orange juice, 1 tablespoon finely chopped parsley, and 3 cloves garlic, finely chopped. Cover and refrigerate till serving time. (There is another recipe for Peach Salsa in the Recipe Index, page 246.)

12. Oatmeal is my favorite morning meal. Serve up a bowl of rolled oats with bananas, strawberries, or any other fresh fruit and you've got plenty of fiber (plus, with some skim milk or rice milk, and a tablespoon of Carnation powdered milk, you've got a dose of calcium first thing in the morning!). And, if the experts at the Food and Drug Administration are right, oatmeal or cold cereal made with rolled oats may even help to reduce heart disease! So eat up!

13. Keep frozen fruit on hand for fast, healthy shakes. Freeze seedless grapes and pop them in your mouth—they're just like candy! Freeze your overripe bananas before they spoil, then blend together 1 frozen banana, 2 frozen strawberries, ½ cup skim milk, and a dash of vanilla. Enjoy!

14. Don't be turned off by things just because they're different. If you try five new vegetables and find one you like, you're already ahead of the game. One of my

discoveries: baby eggplants!—which are rich with their own natural and delicious oils. Sauté and serve with white chestnuts and broccoli over brown rice and you've got a meal. Yum-yum!

15. Instead of deli coleslaw, make delicious jicama slaw. Shred 1 pound jicama; add 1 carrot, peeled and julienned. Combine 1 cup vinegar, 1 bunch chopped chives, ½ cup lime juice, cayenne pepper (lots of it), and 1 teaspoon cilantro, and pour over veggies.

16. For a main course meal, stir-fry together artichokes and mushrooms and roasted peppers. Here's how: Put peppers in the oven and roast till burned black, then remove from heat and put in a covered container and let them "steam" on their own to separate the skin from the flesh. Remove skin and seeds and discard, then add the flesh to cut-up mushrooms and artichokes. Sauté in fresh chicken broth (not the salty commercial kind), along with a touch of garlic, fresh basil, and chopped onion.

17. To make fresh chicken broth, boil several pieces of chicken with bones in water (add an onion for extra flavor); remove chicken and put the water in the refrigerator overnight. In the morning, skim off the fat; then pour broth into 1- or 2-cup containers. Freeze for future use. (Chop the chicken up for a healthy chicken-and-vegetable salad—instead of mayo, use a little nonfat plain yogurt.)

18. Don't mash potatoes with butter, salt, and whole milk and top with sour cream— that's old-fashioned non-Voltage thinking. Instead, try a little low-fat buttermilk for a buttery taste. Or lose the taste of butter altogether and mash them with rice milk or fresh garlic. (For real garlicky mashed potatoes, toss a garlic clove into the boiling water as you're boiling the potatoes. Save the liquid and mash a little in with the potatoes along with a tablespoon of olive oil and black pepper.)

19. To make the most delicious sweet potatoes: Bake, add ginger, a dash of cayenne pepper, and a splash of orange juice. Mash together in a food mill. Do the same with acorn squash or pumpkin, and serve with fish or chicken and a confit of onions (red onion marinated with vinegar and thyme).

20. Cut acorn squash in half, sprinkle with cinnamon and nutmeg, and microwave (covered) for about 8 to 10 minutes for a fast, delicious snack or side dish.

21. Instead of serving baked potatoes with sour cream, cheddar cheese, and bacon, try nonfat yogurt on top . . . or salt-free, low-fat cottage cheese . . . or salsa . . . or fresh, grated horseradish.

22. Turn a baked potato into a lunch with a topping of tuna packed in water . . . or black beans . . . or steamed broccoli florets and ½ teaspoon grated low-sodium cheese and a touch of Mrs. Dash hot pepper mixture.

23. Another potato favorite: salt-free, low-fat cottage cheese and "High Voltage pepper confetti"—that's green, yellow, and red peppers and diced jalapeños, marinated with warm vinegar and lemon juice. Let it sit so the flavors blend together (when you warm the vinegar and pour it over the peppers, it not only tenderizes them, but helps the flavors to saturate).

24. Top sliced baked peaches, pears, or apples with a crumble made from oats, chopped pecans, and 1 teaspoon shredded coconut, 2 tablespoons apple juice or orange juice, cinnamon, and cardamom. Kids love this one (and me too)!

25. Use fresh fruit juices to sauté with extra flavor. Sauté fresh scallops with orange juice and lime juice, then serve over wilted arugula or spinach. (To "wilt," put arugula or spinach in a pan with ¾ cup water; steam till wilted; add scallops and reduce the liquid to a sauce.)

26. For a delicious turkey meatloaf or tasty turkey burgers, add a little chopped onion and Worcestershire sauce and your favorite spices to ground turkey. Or sauté diced onions with garlic, fresh thyme, and parsley. Cool and mix with ground turkey, add pepper and a splash of lemon juice. Make into patties and bake at 350 degrees.

27. Use a teaspoon of any of the all-fruit jams (Polaner apricot, strawberry, and raspberry are my favorites) as a sweetener in plain yogurt or to add some zip to the hot cereal of your choice.

28. To make a delicious "cappuccino" pudding, combine ½ to 1 package Knox gelatin (depending on how firm you like your pudding) with 1 cup skim milk, 1 packet Sweet'n Low, 1 tablespoon instant coffee (or more, depending on how strong a coffee flavor you like), and ice cubes. Blend in blender. Pour pudding mixture into individual cups (you don't want to be tempted to eat the whole bowl!), and freeze. For other flavors, substitute strawberries or bananas for the coffee.

29. Add fresh basil to a salad made from sliced ripe tomatoes, cucumbers, sweet onions, and a little no-salt mozzarella cheese. Season with black pepper and drizzle with a teaspoon of olive oil. Add basil to eggplant, zucchini, or peppers, or to jazz up a salt-free tomato-based sauce or soup.

30. For a special spinach salad, chop in hard-boiled egg, no-salt mozzarella, or crumbled, aged, salt-free goat cheese.

31. Serve up a "rainbow" fruit bowl—half a cantaloupe stuffed with blueberries and raspberries. Serve chilled in a bowl of crushed ice.

32. Get into fiber-rich grains instead of pasta. Cook up a double batch of barley; freeze in 1-cup portions. When ready to use, thaw in the refrigerator or defrost in the microwave. Fluff with a fork and add to soups, stews, salads, and casseroles.

33. Grill skewers of fresh shrimp, mushrooms, slices of green pepper, onions, and tomatoes. Season creatively with black pepper and a dash of cayenne and cumin. Serve with ½ cup couscous.

34. Make and bake healthy potato pancakes: Grate potatoes and onions (to keep them from "blackening"—it happens when the mixture oxidizes—add a few drops of lemon juice). Spice with black pepper, form into patties, and oven-bake at 350 degrees. Serve with homemade applesauce made from Golden Delicious or Granny Smith apples (use apple juice as a sweetener instead of sugar).

35. Core a Rome apple, and stuff with chopped walnuts, dates, prunes, cinnamon, nutmeg, and mace. Pour ½ cup orange juice over it and bake at 350 degrees for

35 minutes covered, then 25 minutes uncovered. Or do it quicker in the microwave!

36. For super curried shrimp for two: Sauté 1 onion till translucent; add a garlic clove and 2 teaspoons curry powder and cook down for about 3 minutes. Toss in sliced zucchini, red and green peppers (1 ½ cups each), 2 cups diced tomatoes, ½ cup chicken stock, and simmer for ten minutes. Toss in 12 shrimp (about 6 per person). Serve over steamed couscous.

37. Slice an eggplant in half; bake and stuff with an assortment of sautéed vegetables and a tablespoon of ricotta cheese (use the low-fat, low-sodium kind).

38. Make your own eggplant caviar: Grill or roast eggplant to remove skin; discard skin and scoop out eggplant; put flesh in a food mill and add lemon juice, cumin, cayenne pepper, olive oil, and blend. Add parsley, oregano, and cilantro, and serve as a dip for crudités, or as a side dish with grilled chicken or fish.

39. Toss some steamed fresh littleneck clams, seasoned with garlic, oregano, rosemary, red pepper flakes, and lemon juice, into a bowl of hot couscous. Add a lot of chopped parsley to give it color and flavor. This can be an elegant meal for entertaining.

40. Stuff a baked no-salt corn tortilla with black beans, corn, and shredded lettuce, chopped tomatoes and onions, and grated no-fat, low-sodium cheese. (Watch out that you don't go back and eat all the tortillas. If you are a "bet you can't eat just one" type, skip this tip.)

41. Use a little yellow cornmeal (add the seasonings of your choice) to add crunchiness and color in a coating for oven-baked chicken or fish. It sure beats Shake'n Bake!

42. Commercial tomato sauces are junk food city (sugar, salt, fat—you don't want to know—or maybe you do!). Check out the new crop of low-sodium (and no-sodium) sauces, find one whose taste you like (or better yet, make your own—

see our recipe, page 244), and spoon over brown rice, couscous, or especially spaghetti squash (which is one of my all-time favorites). If you miss pasta, you'll love this! Use no more than ½ cup sauce.

43. Go wild with all sorts of flavored vinegar—raspberry, red pepper, mint, rosemary, tarragon—not only to add flavor and zest to salads, but to add a tart and wonderful flavor to fish, chicken, and vegetables (important when you're replacing salt!).

44. Serve up baked winter squash topped with shallots, peppers, and a sprinkle of pine nuts; or with a sauce made from sautéed onion, chopped red and green peppers, garlic, and a little diced zucchini, fresh oregano, and fresh thyme. Cover and simmer (25 minutes), and pour over squash. Delicious!

45. Looking for a healthy, easy lunch? Try black beans and corn sliced off the cob (if you must use Niblets, use the frozen-without-salt kind; if canned, rinse to remove as much salt as possible); add chilies and a fresh tomato salad on the side.

46. Add a little mint and a splash of lemon juice to rice; cumin, mint, and cardamom to couscous for a traditional North African flavor; or a splash of olive oil and chopped veggies to bulgur wheat for a quick salad.

47. To flavor brown rice (we're all about flavor big-time!), add a little sautéed onion, garlic cloves, and bay leaf and steam together. Or add onions, diced carrots, celery, and mushrooms as a garnish for eye appeal and texture.

48. Another add-flavor-to-rice tip that one of my clients picked up at Canyon Ranch Spa: For extra flavor, drop a tea bag of your favorite tea in the pot as the rice cooks.

49. Get into the habit of making big pots of soup or chili—meat chili, bean chili, or ground turkey, however you like it (I'm not going to go to war with you over meat, remember. I have bigger battles).

50. Toast wheat germ—it's a nice substitute for finely chopped nuts when you're watching calories.

51. Easy side dishes: Sauté spinach, kale, and broccoli with garlic and no more than 1 tablespoon olive oil (I do it with as little as I can). Sprinkle with lemon and serve. Or make a triple-mushroom sauté: porcini, Portobello, and shiitake mushrooms, with wild rice. Sprinkle with 1 ounce chopped pecans. Sauté sliced yellow squash, zucchini, and mushroom; sprinkle with sesame seeds and serve.

> **Volt-Note!**
>
> For me, going to a restaurant is a social time—to see people, for conversations, to network. Sometimes I eat before I go (I don't always trust the food); and if I haven't eaten beforehand, seldom do I order a full entree. Instead, I share with someone, or take half home; or I order two appetizers or a salad and an appetizer instead of an entree. Of course, this may not be your style, but I live my way because I have to—and I want to. If I didn't, I wouldn't look or feel the way I do. But I really treasure my energy and I **DON'T WANT TO DO ANYTHING TO JEOPARDIZE IT.**

Quick Snacks

1. A banana, clementine, peach, or other sweet fruit.
2. 100-calorie fat-free yogurt.
3. Popcorn (season with garlic, cayenne pepper, cumin powder).
4. Frozen "cookies" (puree fresh fruit in your blender; spoon onto a cookie sheet into cookie-size shapes and freeze).
5. Cut-up veggies and no-salt hummus or salsa.
6. A hard-boiled egg (you can take it anywhere).
7. A baked potato (8 minutes in the microwave); bag it and take it anywhere. I DO THIS A LOT.
8. A bowl of berries.
9. Puffed rice or shredded wheat cereal—portion it into individual bags and eat on the run. Good with or without milk.
10. Rice cake topped with all-fruit jam, 1 teaspoon salt- and sugar-free peanut butter, or salt-free cottage cheese (add an apple and it's practically a meal!).

> **Volt-Note!**
>
> Trade-offs: Some people say that Star Power is expensive. "All those fresh fruits and vegetables," they moan. But listen here: The High Voltage way of eating will also result in more energy, less fatigue, fewer doctor bills in the long run. Making your own dressing from balsamic vinegar and herbs is cheaper than buying bottled dressings (and better-tasting than most of them too). If you're an oatmeal eater, buy it in bulk—nice savings over sugary processed cereal (remember, in addition to your breakfast, you're paying for Tony the Tiger too!).

11. Sugar-free applesauce—mix with plain yogurt, sprinkle with wheat germ for crunch, a touch of cinnamon for extra flavor.
12. A handful of bean sprouts (the crunchy bean part). Bag 'em and grab 'em on the go.
13. 1 ounce of unsalted almonds (I'm saying 1 ounce here—not a 10-ounce bag).

Delete from Consciousness (I Can't Say It Enough)

- Creamy or oily sauces like hollandaise and béarnaise, Alfredo sauce, and pesto.
- Anything fried or sautéed in butter.
- Fatty meats and poultry like pork, spareribs, duck, or goose, and processed luncheon meats.

Volt-Note!

How to Cook it: In general, simple preparations are best. Don't drench food in cheese or butter, coat it with crumbs, or fry it in oils, and you should be fine. Do broil, bake, boil, grill, roast, poach, steam, and fat-free sauté. Fat-free sautéing is done in a skillet over a lower heat than regular sautéing, and with a small amount of liquid (say, broth) or a fat-free cooking spray, as a substitute for butter or oil.

To poach, the food is covered, just barely, in a simmering liquid.

Steaming preserves the nutrients of veggies, fish, or chicken and isn't hard to do. Pour a small amount of water into the pot, place food on a rack above the liquid, cover and heat.

123 Things to Do or Think About Instead of Food

1. Read a book on angels or visit an angel shop.
2. Practice the art of flower arranging.
3. Take singing lessons.
4. Write a letter to a friend you haven't spoken to in a long time.
5. Sign up for a class on herbalism and holistic medicine.
6. Plunge into foreign language study. Then go to where they speak it—and practice your newly acquired ability.
7. Get a pet.
8. Draw your pet.
9. Plant a garden.

10. Improve your tennis game.

11. Have your dreams analyzed.

12. Invite a friend over and give each other facials.

13. Take your child to the library.

14. Read a mystery.

15. Go to the zoo.

16. Find a yoga or tai chi class.

17. Plan a vacation to some exotic locale. Go there.

18. Write down your real feelings about your boss or supervisor (but tear it up before you send it—and if it's on your computer, don't save it!).

19. Paint your kitchen.

20. Clean out your garage.

21. Decide what color your next set of sheets or towels is going to be— check out the local sales.

22. Investigate ballooning.

23. Take flamenco lessons.

24. Volunteer at your local animal shelter—and give a home to a stray.

25. Learn CPR—and practice on a cutie pie.

26. Invite the gang over to talk about whether extraterrestrials really exist— then rent the video *E.T.* Serve salt-free popcorn only.

27. Become a class parent.

28. Make pottery.

29. Drive to the beach and build a sand castle.

30. Knit a six-foot scarf.

31. Have your tea leaves read.

32. Compose a poem for someone special. Get up the courage to give it to him or her.

33. Visit your local "love" shop and check out all the new toys (massage oils, vibrators, edible underwear). Treat yourself—go, girl!

34. Find a charity for your old (too big) clothes.

35. Try on all your old lipsticks and throw away the ones you don't like anymore.

36. Sew a quilt.

37. Register for a course at your high school's adult education department or local college's continuing education.

38. Learn to ski.
39. Go to the library (my mother's favorite hangout). They have everything under the sun there—classes, courses, videos, magazines. Even books . . .
40. Study guitar.
41. Go on-line (or if you don't have a computer, get connected at your nearest cyber-cafe).
42. Go Rollerblading.
43. Recall past lives.
44. Call your mom.
45. Start a journal.
46. Redo your résumé.
47. Refinish your husband's old desk.
48. Indulge in a full-body massage.
49. Change your hair color.
50. Head to your local department store and have your makeup done (be sure to ask for free samples).
51. Research your family tree.
52. Run for the local school board.
53. Sort your family photographs.
54. Learn to sail.
55. Go to clown school.
56. Tweeze your eyebrows—or have them done professionally.
57. Start a home-based business.
58. Collect shells.
59. Write a love letter to your spouse or lover (real or imaginary).
60. Give your lover a foot massage with lavender-scented oil.
61. Sort your earrings.
62. Learn to yodel.
63. Find someone to repair your old watch.
64. Gild a frame and have a mirror put in it.
65. Share the silliest thing you ever did as a kid with your best friend.
66. Volunteer for "Race for the Cure."
67. Try on new eyeglass frames.
68. Shop for a fabulous new nightgown.
69. Raise money for your church.

70. Share a near-death experience with a friend.
71. Stencil your bathroom walls.
72. Save a landmark.
73. Set up a greeting card file.
74. Create your own greeting cards.
75. Spend the afternoon at a museum.
76. Start a book club.
77. Buy a thousand-piece jigsaw puzzle. Don't go to sleep till you're at least half done.
78. Figure out how much money you're saving by not buying fat-free snacks . . . and start a bank account.
79. Take up photography.
80. Plan a yard sale.
81. Write your congressman.
82. Discover tap dancing.
83. Learn to waltz.
84. Bleach your teeth.
85. Go for a walk in the park.
86. Donate your old paperback best-sellers to the local hospital.
87. Decoupage a blanket chest.
88. Go on a house or garden tour.
89. Buy tickets to a concert—rock, jazz, whatever turns you on.
90. Go to a lecture.
91. Give a lecture.
92. Dig out an old paint-by-numbers kit and get into it (get your grandchild to help).
93. Read up on how to make soap . . . then make it.
94. Coordinate a cleanup day for your local park.
95. Paint scenery at your town's little-theater company.
96. Climb a hill and roll down it.
97. Try on wigs.
98. Plant a tree.
99. Go bike riding with a friend.
100. Watch the sunrise. Or the sunset.
101. Pick out new toothbrushes—a different color for every day of the week.

102. Arrange your wardrobe by color and category.
103. Line your dresser drawers with scented paper.
104. Sort your socks and get rid of the odd ones.
105. Get your legs waxed.
106. Make love.
107. Learn how to make slipcovers.
108. Go house hunting.
109. Master horseback riding.
110. Rent a rowboat with your true love.
111. Try Waverunners or Jet Skis.
112. Organize a volleyball game.
113. Take an investment course . . . then invest.
114. Catalog your video library.
115. Start a family newsletter.
116. Form a cousins' club.
117. Try out for the choir.
118. Volunteer to baby-sit for a friend's child one night a week.
119. Attend a channeling session.
120. Choose a crystal for someone you love.
121. Pick out a new room-freshener scent.
122. Join an adult ballet class.
123. Get hypnotized (but don't do anything I wouldn't do . . . which, I realize, doesn't leave out much!).

Backsliding . . . Again

Once you've gotten your weight to a certain point—to goal weight or fairly close—many people tend to relax in their habits a bit. This is a crucial time. If you don't stay close to the scale—keeping daily weigh-ins—all of a sudden, ten pounds will creep back on. When this happens, people are always surprised ("How did this happen?" they say). In these cases, I recommend doing an abbreviated Spa weekend to get you back on track: keeping the food diary, writing everything down, just like you did the first time. As a precaution, I often take people a couple of pounds under where they want to be—so we have a few pounds to play with. Besides, I tell my clients—"Don't get overconfident when people start telling you how wonderful you look. Remember that many people *always* think you look just fine the way you are (like your mother!), and others don't always tell the truth—do you?" Well, I get paid to tell the truth. It may sound brutal to my clients, but they know it's coming from a good place.

ENERGY UP! WHOO!

Chapter 9

WHOO! KEEPING THE ENERGY FLOWING

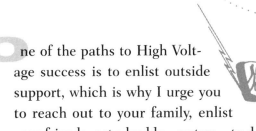

One of the paths to High Voltage success is to enlist outside support, which is why I urge you to reach out to your family, enlist your friends, get a buddy—or two—to do this with you. Form an Energy UP! Club and get together one or two nights a week to share exercise strategies, recipes, and beauty tips that will make this lifestyle work. I always say, get a bunch of like-minded people together, and it reinforces the positive energy flow. Plus, as you see results, you're going to want to find other ways to help each other carry this through.

Forming your own energy group can be especially important if you're isolated in a rural area or small town. Write to big companies asking for healthier, salt-and-sugar-free versions of your favorite foods. Maybe if enough of us do it, it'll make an impact! Get together and request that your local restaurant add Star Power choices to their menus, so you can go there to eat lunch or dinner with friends. (And if they don't—eat and party at home: have everyone bring a Star Power dish!)

Just take it with a sense of humor, people. Make it a game—but never forget that we are serious and we are bucking the system. Still, the only way this will become a lifestyle is to pull others to **GET WITH THE**

PROGRAM! And, if you get a big enough group together, call, write to me c/o my publisher (High Voltage, c/o Putnam, 200 Madison Avenue, New York, NY 10016), or e-mail me at Highvoltage@EnergyUp.com. If I'm traveling nearby, I'll come and give you all a personal energy recharge!

So that's my real mission . . . to make a real change. I do aim high, don't I? But like they say, shoot for the moon and settle with the stars (and you all can be Stars!).

So start sharing the message. Because that's when things can start to change on every level. Remember, it's not a diet, it's a life formula, and if it works for you, I want you to turn other people on to the formula so it works for them too.

So come on board. I'll be out there—dancing, shouting, whooing!—and, I hope, meeting many of you. If you're in the audience at one of my energy concerts, let me know you're there. Stand up straight. Shoulders up, back, and down. Raise your arms. Smile, **BIG-TIME** . . . and shout **"ENERGY UP! WHOOOOO!"**

Power Principles for the Rest of Your Life

Finally, when I work with clients, my goal is to create balance—mind and body. When your life is in balance—when you've acknowledged what's blocking your energy and you are on your way to resolving the issues that are stopping you in life—then and only then can you achieve the self-love that allows you to tune in—to accept and succeed at the rest of my program. The results may be on the outside—an **FF** body (remember, that's *F@#!*ING FIERCE!*)!—but High Voltage works from the inside out.

If you understand that my program is not just about exercise, and about what and how much to eat . . .

If you are ready to create the inner happiness that leads to a fit and healthy lifestyle . . .

Then I am going to ask you to incorporate the following six *power principles* into your life—principles that changed my life, changed my clients' lives, and that I know will change yours.

1. *Choose an Affirmation:* This is key to my program. I want you to start your day with a positive thought, and try to repeat it whenever you can. After all, one crunch or sit-up isn't going to give you great abs; you've got to work at it. So work your affirmation muscle—then and only then will it happen for you.

CAN YOU GO ONE SINGLE DAY **WITHOUT** A NEGATIVE THOUGHT? SOUND SIMPLE? WELL, **TRY IT!**

2. *Choose a Daily Activity:* That activity could be working out to an at-home exercise video; it could be a commitment to go for a brisk daily walk—twenty-five minutes a day to start. Just remember the old saying: your body *is* your temple. Treat it with reverence and respect. Plus, your body is also what carries you around all day. You want to live and play on this planet, you've got to keep your body toned up and tuned in.

3. *Listen to Music That Energizes You:* Rock 'n' roll, classical, country, jazz—the choice is yours (I'm a dance music baby myself). Music is the heartbeat of my program; it's now even understood to have MAJOR healing effects on the emotional system (the more rhythmic the music, the more likely it is to lift your mood). Music can lift you up when you're depressed, calm you down when you're stressed. Why do you think they play elevator music in dentists' offices? Think about it!

4. *Look at Food as Body Fuel:* Realize that what you put into your body is not only what you become, but what you'll get out of it. Food is not love, it is not ecstasy, it is not solace; it is fuel! It is what gives you power—just as gas puts power in your car. So give your body *good fuel!* Feed yourself dead food and you've got a dead body!

5. *Perform an Act of Kindness Once a Day:* Once a day, do something kind for someone. Smile at the woman sitting across from you on the bus. Open the door for someone. If someone cuts you off on the road, instead of yelling **F@#!* YOU!**—yell **BLESS YOU!** It's *amazing* how good you feel when you do something nice for another human being.

6. *Take Private Time:* Most of us are so busy with careers and kids that we forget about the importance of time for ourselves. Read a book. Take a walk. Indulge in a bath by candlelight. Get into the habit of taking time just for you! If you don't do it—if you don't **VALUE** yourself enough to do it—no one will!

This book is about taking charge of your whole life—not just what you eat. You eat in accordance with the way you treat yourself. **IF YOU LOVE YOURSELF, YOU WILL COME TO A POINT WHERE YOU WILL NATURALLY EAT WHAT IS GOOD FOR YOU, WITHOUT HAVING TO THINK ABOUT IT!**

ENERGY UP! WHOO!

P O W E R
S T A T I O N

FREE

YOUR

BODY,

FREE

YOUR

SOUL.

ENER-

GIZE.

TAKE

CONTROL.

HIGH VOLTAGE'S
MONTH OF MENUS

The **High Voltage Maintenance Menu** offers a month of food choices, all based on the **High Voltage Ten Commandments.** Ideally, one's main meal should be at midday; if that is not possible for you, simply reverse the lunch and dinner selections as shown. Unless otherwise indicated, portion size for side order grains and rice are ½ cup; entree sizes are 1 cup; fish, poultry, and meats are 4-to-6-ounce servings; omelets and breakfast eggs are made from 1 egg or 2 egg whites. All sautéing and cooking is done with 1 tablespoon oil per day and with nonstick cooking spray. All nutritional analysis is approximate.

Key for Recipes:

Boldface means the recipe for this dish can be found in the Recipes section, on the page indicated.
*means a description of this dish is in the Fifty-one Food Tips, on the page indicated.

Week I

Day 1 (Sunday)

Rice cake with 1 tablespoon raspberry jam
½ cup fresh citrus salad (oranges, grapefruit,
    tangerine, garnished with mint)
Coffee or tea

Spicy turkey burger with Voltage-baked "fries"*
Cucumber, onion, and tomato salad with **Garlic
    Herb Dressing** (p. 243)
Frozen banana rolled with 1 tablespoon
    chopped nuts and toasted wheat germ

Curried Carrot and Acorn Squash Soup
    (p. 239)
Vegetable lasagna
Whipped Peach Mousse (see Whipped
    Strawberry "Mousse," p. 238)

Day 2 (Monday)

1 poached egg
½ pink grapefruit
Coffee or tea

Tuna taco with shredded veggies and black
    beans
Large green salad with popcorn "croutons"
Red seedless grapes

Swordfish Salad Niçoise (p. 254)
Chopped pepper salad with balsamic vinegar
Crunchy Voltage-baked apple* (p. 214)

Day 3 (Tuesday)

½ cup rolled oats or oatmeal
Fresh mango slices
Coffee or tea

Delicious Tuscan Bean Soup (p. 245)
Romaine lettuce, avocado, and Vidalia onion
    salad with balsamic vinegar
Fresh blueberries and raspberries

Chopped tomato salad with herb vinegar
Golden Crab Cakes (p. 254) with dill-spiked
    yogurt
½ cup of barley tossed with broccoli florets
Frozen applesauce "cookies"* (p. 217)

Day 4 (Wednesday)

Melon wedge
Bran cereal with ½ cup nonfat vanilla yogurt,
    sprinkle of nutmeg
Coffee or tea

Lemon-grilled chicken breast
Bibb lettuce and celery salad with **Lemon-Basil
    Vinaigrette** (p. 237)
Fresh pineapple

Spicy Baked Red Snapper Tacos (p. 255)
Tea-flavored rice* (p. 216)
Cappuccino pudding* (p. 214)

Day 5 (Thursday)

Low-sodium vegetable juice
Rice cake with 1 teaspoon no-salt peanut butter
  and 1 teaspoon all-fruit jam
Melon wedges with mint
Coffee or tea

Greek cucumber salad with nonfat plain yogurt
  and mint
Dannii's Grilled Salmon Tabouli (p. 256)
Pan-seared asparagus with lemon
Fresh kiwi fruit

Voltage Chicken with Vegetables and Couscous
Triple mushroom sauté* (p. 217)
Raspberry-Nectarine Ice (p. 257)

Day 6 (Friday)

Fresh fruit salad
Shredded wheat cereal with no-fat milk
Coffee or tea

Baked potato with **Roasted Corn and Red
  Pepper Salsa** (p. 257)
Large green salad with **Shallot-Mustard
  Vinaigrette** (p. 242)
Slice of honeydew

Poached Scallops with Green Sauce (p. 253)
Roasted and mashed acorn squash with
  cayenne pepper* (p. 212)
Curried Banana (p. 247)

Day 7 (Saturday)

Whole-grain cereal with 2 tablespoons chopped
  apple and cinnamon
Coffee or tea

Chicken salad with vegetables and yogurt
½ cup couscous with mint
Sliced peaches and raspberries

Japanese Restaurant Dinner
Japanese watercress salad
Sushi
Green tea

Week II

Day 8 (Sunday)

Company Brunch
½ pink grapefruit
Fluffy egg-white omelet with fresh vegetables
Chunked potatoes cooked with bell peppers and
  diced onions
Coffee or tea

Cold Asparagus Soup (p. 250)
Tower Tabouli (p. 261)
Red plum or peach

Baby greens with **Roasted Red Pepper
  Vinaigrette** (p. 245)
Curried shrimp* (p. 215) with couscous
Sautéed yellow squash and green zucchini with
  mushrooms and sesame seeds* (p. 217)
Fresh fruit salad

Day 9 (Monday)
Cranberry orange juice
Whole-grain hot cereal with skim milk, dash of
vanilla
Coffee or tea

Roasted Tomato and Garlic Soup (p. 258)
Turkey burger with green salad and balsamic
vinegar
Cantaloupe and honeydew chunks

Arugula, wild mushrooms, and red onion salad
Baked chicken with herbs (remove skin)
Garlic mashed potatoes* (p. 212)
Apple-ginger compote* (p. 214)

Day 10 (Tuesday)
Citrus salad
Rice cake with 1 teaspoon low-fat, no-salt
cottage cheese, dash of cinnamon
Coffee or tea

Spicy Yellow Lentil Stew (p. 258)
Large green salad with rosemary vinegar
100-calorie strawberry-banana yogurt

Salad of greens with chickpeas and wild cherry
vinegar
Oriental Grilled Chicken (p. 259)
Baked Red and Yellow Tomatoes (p. 237)
Poached pears splashed with orange-lime juice

Day 11 (Wednesday)
High Voltage Banana-Strawberry Shake
(p. 259)
Coffee or tea

Spinach salad with hard-boiled egg and no-salt
goat cheese
Plain yogurt swirled with peaches and coconut

Salmon Steak with Citrus Vinaigrette (p. 252)
Fresh corn on the cob
Plain yogurt swirled with 1 tablespoon all-fruit
jam

Day 12 (Thursday)
Oatmeal with fresh fruit, ½ cup rice milk, and ½
teaspoon chopped pecans
Coffee or tea

Fast-Food Lunch
Grilled chicken breast sandwich (remove bun)
Salad bar
Piece of fresh fruit

Roasted Rosemary Lamb (p. 260)
Boiled new potatoes with parsley and herbs
Sautéed Spinach and Leeks (p. 256)
Whipped Banana Mousse (see Whipped
Strawberry "Mousse," p. 238)

Day 13 (Friday)
Orange slices
Onion-basil egg-white omelet with 1 ounce
grated low-salt cheese
Coffee or tea

Baked potato pancakes* (p. 214) with sugar-
free applesauce
Large green salad with **Garlic Herb Dressing**
(p. 243)
Peach

Herb-roasted chicken
Baked sweet potatoes
Lemon-sautéed kale, spinach, and mushrooms
Air-popped popcorn sprinkled with onion
powder

Day 14 (Saturday)
Rainbow fruit bowl filled with berries* (p. 214)
Coffee or tea

Refreshing Chilled Cucumber-Basil Soup
(p. 242)
½ cup cumin-mint-cardamom couscous
Nectarine

Green salad with blueberry vinegar
**Pan-Roasted Monkfish with Wild Mushroom
Ragout** (p. 236)
Cantaloupe half, filled with berries

Week III

Day 15 (Sunday)
Citrus salad
Fluffy tomato-basil omelet
Coffee or tea

Summer Squash Bisque (p. 260)
**6-Vegetable Terrine with Peppered Fresh
Tomato Sauce** (p. 240)
Fresh blackberries and orange wedges

Mixed greens with balsamic vinegar
Energy Antipasto Dinner (p. 251)
Wild rice
Peach sorbet

Day 16 (Monday)
High Voltage Spa "Morning Sunrise" shake
(p. 196)
Coffee or tea

Tuna niçoise (water-packed tuna, string beans,
hard-boiled egg slices, boiled potato on
mixed green salad with balsamic vinegar)
Vanilla yogurt with 1 tablespoon chopped raisins
and dates

Broiled catfish
Rosemary and buttermilk mashed potatoes*
(p. 212)
Sautéed snow peas and carrots
Strawberries, yogurt, and granola parfait

Day 17 (Tuesday)
Orange and grapefruit slices
Hard-boiled egg
Coffee or tea

Green salad with tomatoes, no-salt mozzarella,
and blueberry vinegar

Dungeon Dungeness Crab Salad (p. 261)
Baked potato with grated fresh horseradish
Frozen grapes

Italian Vegetable Frittata (p. 246)
Sesame green beans with zucchini and red
    peppers
Sliced peaches with strawberries

Day 18 (Wednesday)

Spanish egg scramble (scrambled eggs with
    green chilies and low-salt cheese)
Fresh fruit salad
Coffee or tea

Green salad with **Red Onion Dressing** (p. 248)
Vegetarian Chili (p. 262)
Frozen banana

Large green salad with purple basil vinegar
Southwestern-Style Turkey Cassoulet
    (p. 262)
Steamed vegetables
Watermelon

Day 19 (Thursday)

High Voltage tofu-berry shake
Tangerine
Coffee or tea

Baked potato with salsa* (p. 213)
Green salad with cucumbers, carrots, celery,
    cherry tomatoes, and balsamic vinaigrette

Grilled skewered shrimp with onions, peppers
    and tomatoes
Seasoned brown rice* (p. 216)
Grapefruit ice

Day 20 (Friday)

Oatmeal with cinnamon and sliced oranges
Coffee or tea

Golden Crab Cakes (p. 254)
Fresh tomatoes, cucumbers, and red peppers
Clementines

Casual Dinner Party
Eggplant "caviar" appetizers* (p. 215)
Crudités with yogurt dip
Turkey chili (ground turkey with chopped
    tomatoes, nonfat sour cream, and shredded
    low-sodium cheese)
Grated red-cabbage and Carrot Slaw
Seasoned vegetable chips* (p. 209)
Fresh fruit platter

Day 21 (Saturday)

Hot whole-wheat cereal
Mango slices
Coffee or tea

Citrus-Grilled Turkey Salad (p. 263)
Jicama slaw* (p. 212)
Fresh cherries

Herb-roasted chicken
New potatoes with rosemary

233

Steamed asparagus with lemon and tarragon
Poached pears

Week IV

Day 22 (Sunday)

Rice cake with 1 tablespoon low-fat, no-salt
    cottage cheese, cinnamon, and nutmeg
Grapefruit half
Coffee or tea

Scallops poached in lime juice* (p. 213)
Onion and Pineapple Salsa (p. 264)
Steamed Wheatberries
Green seedless grapes

Green salad with blueberry-orange mint vinegar
Shrimp on a bed of steamed broccoli rabe
Oven-dried tomatoes
Fresh peach sorbet with white grape juice
    sweetener

Day 23 (Monday)

Yogurt with ¾ cup sugar-free granola and fruit
Coffee or tea

Chicken corn chowder
Roasted and mashed squash with cinnamon
    and nutmeg
Vanilla yogurt with blueberries

Sliced cucumber, radish, and green onions with
    rice-wine vinegar
Grilled Tuna with Chickpeas and Spinach
    (p. 241)
Orange wedges

Day 24 (Tuesday)

Oatmeal with sliced banana and almond milk
    sprinkled with cinnamon
Coffee or tea

Green salad with nasturtium vinegar
Spaghetti squash with **Tomato Sauce with
    Mushrooms** (p. 244)
Fresh papaya

Baked chicken with **Onion and Pineapple
    Salsa** (p. 264)
Sautéed escarole with garlic and white beans
Whipped Strawberry "Mousse" (p. 238)

Day 25 (Wednesday)

"Berry Nice" breakfast shake (fresh berries,
    orange juice, banana, and vanilla yogurt in
    blender)
Coffee or tea

Broiled turkey burgers
Steamed couscous
Fresh apple-pear sauce

Lettuce, onions, and cucumbers with tarragon
    dressing
Vegetarian Chili (p. 262)
Baked sweet potatoes
Fresh fruit salad

Day 26 (Thursday)

Scrambled eggs with diced tomato and low-salt
    grated cheese

Sliced pears
Coffee or tea

Baby eggplant steamed with broccoli and water
    chestnuts* (p. 212)
Brown rice
Pomegranate half and mandarin oranges

Scallion-Shrimp Pancakes (p. 238)
Cayenne-seasoned broccoli and cauliflower
Yogurt parfait

Day 27 (Friday)

Fresh fruit salad
½ cup low-fat, no-salt cottage cheese
Coffee or tea

Green salad with grilled swordfish chunks and
    red peppers
Fresh strawberries

Green salad with **Lemon-Basil Vinaigrette**
    (p. 237)
**Tenderloin of Beef L'Orange with brown rice
    and broccoli** (p. 264)

Day 28 (Saturday)

Rolled oats
Sliced fruit, rice milk, and cinnamon
Coffee or tea

Savory turkey meatloaf* (p. 213) with red
    tomato coulis* (see onion coulis, p. 210)
Basmati rice with onions, carrots, celery, and
    mushrooms
Whipped Raspberry Mousse (see Whipped
    Strawberry "Mousse," p. 238)

Company Dinner
Baked red snapper
Grilled fennel
New potatoes sautéed with black peppercorns
Frozen iced tea

RECLPES

Pan-Roasted Monkfish with Wild Mushroom Ragout

4 SERVINGS

- 4 monkfish (6 ounces each)
- ⅛ teaspoon cayenne pepper
- ¼ teaspoon chili powder
- ¼ teaspoon black pepper
- ¼ teaspoon cumin
- 2 teaspoons rosemary
- 2 teaspoons olive oil

In a large bowl, place monkfish, seasonings, and oil to marinate for 30 minutes.

- 2 teaspoons olive oil
- 1 pound shiitake mushrooms
- 1 pound cremini mushrooms
- 1 pound portobello mushrooms
- 1 pound oyster mushrooms
- 3 garlic cloves, chopped
- 4 shallots, sliced
- ½ teaspoon fresh thyme
- ½ teaspoon chives
- ½ teaspoon parsley
- ¼ cup white wine vinegar

In a skillet, sauté in oil mushrooms, garlic, shallots, and herbs. Cook for 15 minutes. Add monkfish and vinegar. Cover and simmer for 25 minutes. Adjust seasoning.

PER SERVING: ABOUT 301 CAL(ORIES), 34G PRO(TEIN), 26G CAR(BOHYDRATES), 9G FAT, 25% CAL(ORIES) FROM FAT, 43MG CHOL(ESTEROL), 51MG SOD(IUM), 5G FIBER.

Baked Red and Yellow Tomatoes

6 SERVINGS

- 3 garlic cloves, chopped
- 2 shallots, chopped
- 1 teaspoon oregano, chopped
- 1 teaspoon rosemary, chopped
- 1 teaspoon thyme, chopped
- 4 teaspoons basil, chopped
- 1 teaspoon black pepper
- 2 tablespoons lemon juice
- 3 red tomatoes
- 3 yellow tomatoes

Preheat oven to 325°F.

In a small bowl, combine all ingredients except tomatoes; mix well. Cut off ¼ inch of tomato bottom. Add herb mixture to each tomato. Bake for 20 minutes.

PER SERVING: ABOUT 44 CAL, 1G PRO, 11G CAR, 0G FAT, 0% CAL FROM FAT, 0MG CHOL, 13MG SOD, 2G FIBER.

Lemon-Basil Vinaigrette

3 SERVINGS

- ¼ cup diced shallots
- ¼ cup lemon juice
- ⅛ cup orange juice
- ½ cup chopped basil
- 3 teaspoons salt-free mustard
- 2 teaspoons lemon zest
- ¼ teaspoon white pepper

In a small bowl, combine all ingredients; whisk well. Adjust seasoning to taste.

PER SERVING: (2 TEASPOONS): ABOUT 23 CAL, 1G PRO, 6G CAR, 0G FAT, 0% CAL FROM FAT, 65MG CHOL, 2MG SOD, 0G FIBER.

Whipped Strawberry "Mousse"

2 SERVINGS

- 1 cup very cold skim milk
- 1 cup fresh strawberries, cut in ½-inch pieces
- 1 teaspoon vanilla extract

In a medium bowl, with electric beater or hand blender, whip milk about 1 minute (or until triple in volume). Add strawberries and vanilla extract and whip another 30 seconds; pour into dessert goblets. Chill several hours before serving.

PER SERVING: ABOUT 67 CAL, 5G PRO, 11G CAR, 1G FAT, 6% CAL FROM FAT, 2MG CHOL, 64MG SOD, 2G FIBER.

VARIATION: SUBSTITUTE 1 CUP SLICED PEACHES OR OTHER FRESH FRUIT FOR STRAWBERRIES.

Scallion-Shrimp Pancakes

6 SERVINGS (6 PANCAKES)

- 1 cup rice flour
- 3 teaspoons cornstarch
- 1 cup cold water
- 2 whole eggs, beaten
- 4 scallions, thinly sliced
- 2 teaspoons chopped cilantro
- 1 teaspoon minced fresh ginger
  Fresh black pepper to taste
- ½ pound cooked medium shrimp, cleaned, cut lengthwise in half
- 2 teaspoons peanut oil

In a mixing bowl, combine all ingredients except shrimp. Blend well, until the consistency of pancake batter. If mixture is too thick, thin with water, one drop at a time. Fold in shrimp.

Brush a nonstick skillet with peanut oil; heat over medium heat. Ladle ¼ cup batter into hot pan. Cook for 1 to 2 minutes until done. Reserve on warm plate.

PER SERVING: ABOUT 177 CAL, 12G PRO, 23G CAR, 4G FAT, 19% CAL FROM FAT, 135MG CHOL, 127MG SOD, 1G FIBER.

Sautéed Zucchini

4 SERVINGS

4 zucchini, halved lengthwise
2 teaspoons chopped lemon grass
2 teaspoons chopped parsley
2 teaspoons minced garlic
1 teaspoon minced ginger
Cilantro (optional)

In a medium nonstick skillet, sauté zucchini with all ingredients. Cook until zucchini is tender. Top with fresh cilantro if desired.

PER SERVING: About 21 cal, 2g pro, 4g car, 0g fat, 0% cal from fat, 0mg chol, 4mg sod, 2g fiber.

Curried Carrot and Acorn Squash Soup

8 SERVINGS

2 teaspoons olive oil
½ cup diced onion
⅓ cup diced celery
5 teaspoons curry powder
1 pound carrots, diced
1 pound acorn squash, diced
2 quarts water
1 teaspoon chopped ginger
⅛ teaspoon ground cloves
¼ teaspoon ground nutmeg
Plain yogurt, for garnish

In a medium saucepan, heat oil. Add onion, celery, and curry powder. Sauté for 5 minutes over medium heat. Add carrots, squash, and water; bring to a boil. Lower heat, cover, and cook for 30 minutes. Add spices. Garnish with plain yogurt.

PER SERVING: About 53 cal, 1g pro, 11g car, 1g fat, 20% cal from fat, 0mg chol, 23mg sod, 2g fiber.

6-Vegetable Terrine with Peppered Fresh Tomato Sauce

6 TO 7 SERVINGS

10 plum tomatoes, diced
½ teaspoon black pepper, divided
¼ cup balsamic vinegar
3 Japanese eggplants, sliced
1 red bell pepper, quartered
1 yellow bell pepper, quartered
1 green bell pepper, quartered
2 zucchini, sliced
2 leeks, sliced
2 teaspoons rosemary
2 teaspoons thyme
¼ teaspoon garlic powder
1 tablespoon olive oil

For tomato sauce:

Preheat oven to 350°F. Roast tomatoes for 25 minutes.

In food processor, place roasted tomatoes, ¼ teaspoon black pepper, and balsamic vinegar. Set aside.

In a large bowl, combine vegetables. Mix spices, remaining ¼ teaspoon black pepper, and oil. Grill each vegetable, then layer vegetables in a deep baking dish. Cover and bake for 30 minutes. Let cool, then slice. Serve with tomato sauce.

PER SERVING: ABOUT 100 CAL, 3G PRO, 19G CAR, 3G FAT, 21% CAL FROM FAT, 0MG CHOL, 16MG SOD, 6G FIBER.

Grilled Tuna with Chickpeas and Spinach

3 SERVINGS

3 tuna steaks (4 to 6 ounces each)
⅛ teaspoon cayenne pepper
¼ teaspoon ginger
¼ teaspoon cumin

In a large bowl, combine tuna and spices; marinade for at least 1 hour. Grill tuna on each side for 4 minutes, for medium rare to medium done.

2 teaspoons olive oil
1 medium onion, diced
2 garlic cloves, chopped
4 teaspoons curry powder
1 cup coconut milk*
10 ounces spinach
10 ounces cooked chickpeas, rinsed
1 teaspoon black pepper
1 teaspoon cinnamon

In a medium pot, heat oil. Sauté onion, garlic, and curry powder for 5 minutes. Add coconut milk, spinach, chickpeas, black pepper, and cinnamon. Cook for 20 minutes. Adjust seasoning.

PER SERVING: ABOUT 424 CAL,* 30G PRO, 28G CAR, 23G FAT, 47% CAL FROM FAT, 32MG CHOL, 89MG SOD, 2G FIBER.

*Note: 184 of these calories per serving are from coconut milk. We recommend lite coconut milk for a lower calorie count.

241

Shallot-Mustard Vinaigrette

4 SERVINGS

¼ cup diced shallots
¼ cup salt-free mustard
1 teaspoon black pepper
⅛ cup red wine vinegar
⅛ cup balsamic vinegar
Chopped tarragon to taste

In a medium bowl, combine shallots, mustard, and black pepper. Slowly whisk wine and balsamic vinegars into shallot mixture. Add chopped tarragon. Adjust seasoning.

PER SERVING (1 TEASPOON): ABOUT 20 CAL, 1G PRO, 3G CAR, 1G FAT, 26% CAL FROM FAT, 0MG CHOL, 1MG SOD, 0G FIBER.

Refreshing Chilled Cucumber-Basil Soup

4 TO 5 SERVINGS

3 cups plain no-fat yogurt (100 calories per cup)
1 medium cucumber, peeled, grated, coarsely chopped
½ cup chopped fresh basil leaves
4 tablespoons lemon juice
2 garlic cloves, crushed
Ground black pepper to taste
1 cup water

In a large bowl, combine yogurt, cucumber, basil, lemon juice, garlic and pepper. Add water to desired consistency, about 1 cup. Refrigerate at least 1 hour before serving.

PER SERVING: ABOUT 96 CAL, 9G PRO, 15G CAR, 0G FAT, 0% CAL FROM FAT, 2MG CHOL, 107MG SOD, 1G FIBER.

Garlic
Herb Dressing

3 SERVINGS

- 3 teaspoons olive oil
- 6 garlic cloves, chopped
- 4 teaspoons salt-free mustard
- ¼ cup balsamic vinegar
- 2 teaspoons rosemary, chopped
- 2 teaspoons thyme, chopped
- 2 teaspoons parsley, chopped
- 2 teaspoons tarragon, chopped

In a small skillet, over medium heat, heat oil. Add garlic. Simmer until garlic is light brown in color. Place in bowl to cool. Whisk in mustard, vinegar, and herbs.

PER SERVING (2 TEASPOONS): ABOUT 56 CAL, 1G PRO, 4G CAR, 5G FAT, 73% CAL FROM FAT, 0MG CHOL, 2MG SOD, 0G FIBER.

Brown Rice with
Lemon-Pepper Relish

6 SERVINGS

- 3 cups brown rice, cooked (with bay leaf and clove added)
- 1 poblano pepper
- 1 red bell pepper
- 1 yellow bell pepper
- 1 Vidalia onion
- 1 red onion
- 4 teaspoons lemon juice
- ¼ cup orange juice
- 2 teaspoons cilantro

Place peppers in a pan and broil until skin turns black. Remove burned skin. Dice peppers and onions; add lemon juice, orange juice, and cilantro. Serve alongside ½ cup cooked rice per person.

PER SERVING: ABOUT 143 CAL, 3G PRO, 31G CAR, 1G FAT, 6% CAL FROM FAT, 0MG CHOL, 4MG SOD, 3G FIBER.

Tomato Sauce with Mushrooms

4 TO 6 SERVINGS

1 pound ripe tomatoes (10 to 12), peeled and seeded

2 tablespoons olive oil

1 large onion, diced

⅛ cup rice-wine vinegar

1 tablespoon fresh thyme leaves

3 garlic cloves, chopped

½ cup water

8 ounces mushrooms, washed and sliced

½ tablespoon fresh oregano

½ cup chopped basil

White pepper to taste

To peel tomatoes: In a large pan, bring water to boil. Prepare a large bowl of water and ice (ice bath) and set aside. Score each tomato with sharp knife and dip each in boiling water. Remove promptly and place in ice bath. Remove skin. Cut in half. Squeeze to remove seeds.

In a medium-large saucepan, heat 1 tablespoon olive oil, sauté onion until tender and transparent. Add vinegar, thyme leaves, and garlic. Cook for 3 minutes. Add tomatoes and ½ cup water. Simmer 20 to 30 minutes, covered. Remove from heat. Blend in Cuisinart.

In same pan, heat remaining 1 tablespoon oil, sauté mushrooms rapidly. Add to tomato sauce with fresh oregano, basil, and white pepper.

PER SERVING: ABOUT 81 CAL, 2G PRO, 10G CAR, 5G FAT, 48% CAL FROM FAT, 0MG CHOL, 9MG SOD, 2G FIBER.

Roasted Red Pepper Vinaigrette

6 SERVINGS

4 large red bell peppers
¼ cup rice-wine vinegar
¼ cup white wine vinegar
4 teaspoons lemon juice
1 teaspoon white pepper

Preheat broiler.

In a pan, broil peppers until skin turns black. Place in covered container until cool, then wash away burned skin.

In blender, on medium speed, process red bell peppers. Slowly add rice-wine and white wine vinegars, lemon juice, and white pepper. Adjust seasoning.

PER SERVING: (3 TEASPOONS): ABOUT 17 CAL, 0G PRO, 5G CAR, 0G FAT, 0% CAL FROM FAT, 0MG CHOL, 1MG SOD, 1G FIBER.

Delicious Tuscan Bean Soup

10 SERVINGS

1 pound cannellini beans
2 teaspoons olive oil
1 cup diced onion
1 cup diced celery
8 garlic cloves, minced
½ cup diced carrots
3 quarts water
2 cups diced zucchini
2 large tomatoes, diced
2 bay leaves
3 teaspoon fresh rosemary
¼ cup white wine vinegar
Chopped basil, for garnish

In a medium bowl, soak beans in cold water overnight; drain. In a large pot, heat oil. Add onion, celery, garlic, and carrots. Sauté for 5 minutes. Add beans and water; bring to a boil. Cover and simmer slowly for 45 minutes. Then add zucchini, tomatoes, bay leaves, and rosemary. Cook 20 minutes longer. Add vinegar. Garnish with chopped basil.

PER SERVING: ABOUT 184 CAL, 12G PRO, 33G CAR, 1G FAT, 7% CAL FROM FAT, 0MG CHOL, 22MG SOD, 8G FIBER.

Italian Vegetable Frittata

4 SERVINGS

4 egg whites
Nonstick cooking spray
1 Portobello mushroom, chopped
1 small zucchini, chopped
1 small red bell pepper, sliced
1 small tomato, chopped
5 basil leaves, chopped
2 teaspoons fresh oregano
⅛ teaspoon black pepper
2 teaspoons olive oil
⅓ cup low-fat ricotta cheese

Preheat oven to 325°F.

In a medium bowl, beat egg whites until stiff peaks form. Set aside. In a sauté pan, with nonstick cooking spray, place mushroom, zucchini, red bell pepper, tomato, black pepper, and herbs and sauté for 10 minutes. In a separate pan, heat oil; add egg whites. Add sautéed vegetables and ricotta cheese. Bake for 15 minutes.

PER SERVING: ABOUT 69 CAL, 6G PRO, 4G CAR, 3G FAT, 39% CAL FROM FAT, 8MG CHOL, 152MG SOD, 1G FIBER.

Peach Salsa

4 SERVINGS

4 medium peaches, chopped
½ cup chopped green bell pepper
½ cup chopped red onion
3 tablespoons lemon juice
4 tablespoons orange juice
2 tablespoons finely chopped parsley
3 garlic cloves, finely chopped

In a medium bowl, combine all ingredients. Cover and refrigerate until serving time. Serve slightly chilled or at room temperature with grilled chicken.

PER SERVING: ABOUT 47 CAL, 1G PRO, 12G CAR, 0G FAT, 0% CAL FROM FAT, 0MG CHOL, 1MG SOD, 1G FIBER.

Curried Banana

4 SERVINGS

1 cup coconut milk*
1 teaspoon curry powder
Pinch nutmeg
Pinch cinnamon
Pinch ground ginger
Pinch cardamom
4 bananas
½ cup toasted coconut, garnish

Infuse coconut milk with curry powder, nutmeg, cinnamon, ginger, and cardamom. Reduce to half.

Cut bananas on bias. Spoon coconut milk over bananas and glaze under broiler. Garnish with toasted coconut.

PER SERVING: ABOUT 206 CAL,* 2G PRO, 21G CAR, 15G FAT, 59% CAL FROM FAT, 0MG CHOL, 10MG SOD, 2G FIBER.

*Note: We use lite coconut milk for a lower-calorie version.

Peppery Corn Chowder

8 SERVINGS

1 tablespoon olive oil
1 cup diced onion
½ cup diced celery
½ cup diced red bell pepper
½ cup diced green bell pepper
3 cups diced potato
6 cups corn kernels
2 bay leaves
1 teaspoon cayenne pepper
1 teaspoon black pepper
¼ teaspoon nutmeg
1½ quarts water

In a large pot, heat oil. Sauté onion, celery, and red and green bell peppers for 5 minutes. Add potato, corn, and all spices. Simmer for 5 more minutes. Add water and bring to a rapid boil. Cover pot and lower heat to medium. Cook for 35 minutes. Adjust seasoning.

PER SERVING: ABOUT 218 CAL, 6G PRO, 40G CAR, 5G FAT, 21% CAL FROM FAT, 0MG CHOL, 14MG SOD, 5G FIBER.

Red Onion Dressing

6 SERVINGS

1 large red onion, diced in small pieces
2 teaspoons salt-free mustard
1 teaspoon black pepper
¼ cup orange juice
¼ cup red wine vinegar
4 teaspoons chopped cilantro
2 teaspoons thyme

In a bowl, blend onion, mustard, and black pepper. Slowly whisk in orange juice and red wine vinegar. Add cilantro and thyme. Adjust seasoning.

PER SERVING (3 TEASPOONS): ABOUT 16 CAL, 0G PRO, 4G CAR, 0G FAT, 0% CAL FROM FAT, 0MG CHOL, 22MG SOD, 1G FIBER.

Mixed Berries with Scarlet Strawberry Sauce

4 SERVINGS

1 cup blueberries
1 cup blackberries
1 cup raspberries
Juice of 1 lemon
4 to 6 ounces frozen strawberries

In a large bowl, combine blueberries, blackberries, and raspberries. Add lemon juice. Place in individual dessert cups and set aside to chill.

In blender, whirl strawberries until smooth. Drizzle berries in strawberry sauce to serve.

PER SERVING: ABOUT 87 CAL, 1G PRO, 22G CAR, 1G FAT, 5% CAL FROM FAT, 0MG CHOL, 3MG SOD, 5G FIBER.

Voltage Chicken with Vegetables and Couscous

4 SERVINGS

- 2 teaspoons olive oil
- 1 large onion, diced
- 6 garlic cloves, minced
- 3 carrots, cut into ½-inch-thick slices
- 6 ounces skinless, boneless chicken thighs, cut into ½-inch chunks
- 1½ teaspoons curry powder
- 1 teaspoon ground ginger
- ¼ teaspoon cinnamon
- ¼ teaspoon cayenne pepper
- ¼ teaspoon ground allspice
- ½ teaspoon freshly ground black pepper
- 1 yellow summer squash, halved lengthwise and cut into ½-inch slices
- 1 zucchini, halved lengthwise and cut into ½-inch-thick slices
- 1 cup salt-free chicken broth, defatted
- ½ cup water
- ⅔ cup couscous
- ¼ cup chopped fresh cilantro

In a large nonstick skillet, over medium heat, heat olive oil. Add onion and garlic and cook about 5 to 7 minutes, stirring frequently, until onion is softened. Stir in carrots and cook about 2 minutes, stirring frequently.

Add chicken and cook about 2 minutes, until chicken is no longer pink. Add curry powder, ginger, cinnamon, cayenne pepper, allspice, and black pepper and cook about 1 minute, stirring constantly. Add squash, zucchini, broth, and water; bring to boil. Add couscous and cook about 5 minutes longer, stirring frequently, until liquid is absorbed and chicken is cooked through. Stir in cilantro and serve.

PER SERVING: ABOUT 213 CAL, 15G PRO, 31G CAR, 5G FAT, 18% CAL FROM FAT, 28MG CHOL, 45MG SOD, 6G FIBER.

Crunchy Raw Vegetable Slaw

10 SERVINGS

¼ head green cabbage
¼ head red cabbage
2 medium carrots, sliced
1 medium onion
1 cucumber
1 apple
1 yellow bell pepper
3 ripe avocados
2 tablespoons lime juice
2 tablespoons lemon juice
½ teaspoon cumin
4 teaspoons dill, chopped
1 garlic clove, chopped
¼ cup white wine vinegar

In a large bowl, slice green and red cabbages, carrots, onion, cucumber, apple, and yellow bell pepper in very fine pieces. Set aside. Peel and seed avocados. Mash avocado until smooth; combine lime and lemon juices, cumin, dill, and garlic. Combine avocado with sliced vegetables. Add vinegar. Let marinate for 2 hours. Serve.

PER SERVING (4 OUNCES): ABOUT 111 CAL, 2G PRO, 13G CAR, 7G FAT, 52% CAL FROM FAT, 0MG CHOL, 18MG SOD, 3G FIBER.

Cold Asparagus Soup

8 SERVINGS

3 pounds asparagus
2 teaspoons olive oil
1 cup diced onion
½ cup diced celery
2 cups diced potatoes
1 teaspoon white pepper
3½ quarts water, divided into 1 ½ quarts and 2 quarts
1 pint plain yogurt
3 tablespoons white wine vinegar

Wash asparagus. Cut and save about ½ pound asparagus tips for garnish later.

In a medium pot, heat oil. Sauté asparagus, onion, celery, potatoes, and pepper for 10 minutes. Add 1½ quarts water, bring to rapid boil. Lower heat and cover. Cook for 25 minutes.

In food processor, place soup; blend, and strain liquid. Add yogurt and vinegar; mix. Chill for 2 hours.

Fill a large pot with 2 quarts water and bring to a boil. Add asparagus tips and cook for 1 minute. Drain; place tips into ice bath. When cool, drain. Slice asparagus tips lengthwise and use for garnish.

PER SERVING: ABOUT 110 CAL, 5G PRO, 17G CAR, 3G FAT, 25% CAL FROM FAT, 7MG CHOL, 37MG SOD, 3G FIBER.

Energy
Antipasto Dinner

4 SERVINGS

- ¾ pound small red potatoes, quartered
- 1 can (9 ounces) artichoke hearts
- 1 tablespoon extra-virgin olive oil, divided
- 1 medium red onion, cut into 1-inch pieces
- 1 red bell pepper, cut into 1-inch pieces
- 1 yellow bell pepper, cut into 1-inch pieces
- 2 garlic cloves, diced
- 1 zucchini, cut into 1-inch-by-½-inch strips
- 1 cup canned chickpeas, drained and well rinsed
- 4 ounces turkey, cut into 1½-by-½-inch strips
- 3 tablespoons balsamic vinegar
- 1 tablespoon chopped fresh parsley

In a large nonstick skillet, cook potatoes in boiling water for 10 minutes. Add artichokes and continue cooking about 5 minutes. Drain potatoes and artichokes well and pat dry with paper towels. Set aside.

In a small skillet over medium heat, heat 2 teaspoons olive oil. Add onion, bell peppers, and garlic and cook, stirring frequently, about 5 minutes. Stir in potatoes and artichokes and cook about 5 minutes longer. Stir in zucchini and cook, stirring frequently, about 3 minutes, until zucchini is tender but crisp. Stir in chickpeas and turkey and cook about 3 minutes. Gently stir in remaining teaspoon olive oil, vinegar, and parsley. Serve.

PER SERVING: ABOUT 254 CAL, 12G PRO, 41G CAR, 6G FAT, 21% CAL FROM FAT, 15MG CHOL, 262MG SOD, 9G FIBER.

Salmon Steak
with Citrus Vinaigrette

4 SERVINGS

    4 salmon steaks
    ¼ teaspoon cumin
    ¼ teaspoon cayenne pepper
    2 teaspoons fresh thyme
    1 tablespoon orange zest

In a bowl, combine all ingredients; marinate. Set aside for at least one hour.

    2 orange segments
    1 grapefruit segment
    ¼ cup diced red bell pepper
    ¼ cup sliced scallions
    4 teaspoons cilantro
    2 garlic cloves
    ⅛ teaspoon cayenne pepper
    4 teaspoons mint, chopped

In a large bowl, mix all eight ingredients for vinaigrette. Set aside.

Nonstick cooking spray

In a sauté pan, with nonstick cooking spray, sauté salmon for 15 minutes. Top salmon with citrus vinegar.

PER SERVING: ABOUT 628 CAL, 31G PRO, 136G CAR, 2G FAT, 3% CAL FROM FAT, 0MG CHOL, 29MG SOD, 23G FIBER

St. Tropez
Vegetables

6 SERVINGS

    1 large acorn squash
    2 zucchini
    3 tomatoes
    3 large shallots
    2 Japanese eggplants
    1 tablespoon olive oil
    1 teaspoon rosemary
    1 teaspoon thyme
    ⅛ teaspoon cumin
    Juice of 1 lemon

Preheat oven to 375°.

Slice all vegetables ¼-inch thick. Set aside. In a large bowl, combine olive oil, rosemary, thyme, cumin, and lemon juice. Add vegetables and toss together. Place vegetables in parchment paper in sheet pan. Bake for 25 minutes.

PER SERVING: ABOUT 103 CAL, 3G PRO, 20G CAR, 3G FAT, 21% CAL FROM FAT, 0MG CHOL, 14MG SOD, 4G FIBER.

Poached Scallops
with Green Sauce

3 SERVINGS

12 ounces sea scallops
⅛ teaspoon cayenne pepper
1 teaspoon lemon zest
¼ teaspoon nutmeg

In a medium-sized bowl, combine sea scallops with pepper, lemon zest, and nutmeg; marinate for at least 1 hour.

2 cups spinach
1 cup watercress
½ cup basil
½ cup parsley
3 teaspoons tarragon
2 teaspoons thyme
2 tablespoons white wine vinegar
2 tablespoons rice-wine vinegar

For sauce: Steam all greens and herbs together for 5 minutes, then place in blender; mix. Add white wine vinegar and rice-wine vinegar slowly, then place mixture in a sauté pan. Add scallops and simmer for 10 minutes. Adjust seasoning.

PER SERVING: About 110 cal, 20g pro, 5g car, 1g fat, 8% cal from fat, 37mg chol, 208mg sod, 1g fiber.

Emerald Rice

6 SERVINGS

1½ cups white rice
2½ cups water
1 bay leaf
1 clove
1 cinnamon stick
1½ bunches fresh spinach
¼ teaspoon nutmeg

In a large bowl, wash rice in cold water; drain. In a medium pot, place rice, water, bay leaf, clove, and cinnamon stick. Cook for 25 minutes. In another pot, steam spinach for 5 minutes.

In food processor, process spinach and nutmeg. Then mix with rice. Adjust seasoning.

PER SERVING: About 171 cal, 4g pro, 37g car, 0g fat, 0% cal from fat, 0mg chol, 10mg sod, 1g fiber.

Swordfish Salad Niçoise

3 TO 4 SERVINGS

- 1½ pounds swordfish steaks (or use tuna steaks if fresher)
- 1 tablespoon olive oil
- ½ lemon

Rub steaks with olive oil and lemon. Grill and cut into bite-sized pieces.

- ¼ cup olive oil
- ¼ cup balsamic vinegar
- 2 hard-boiled eggs, sliced
- 3 plum tomatoes, quartered
- ¼ pound green beans, steamed
- ¼ pound boiled red potatoes, quartered
- ½ cup fresh herbs such as basil, tarragon, oregano
  Salad greens
  Edible flowers (optional)

In a large bowl, mix olive oil and balsamic vinegar to make a dressing. Toss with all ingredients and arrange artfully on an platter. Sprinkle with edible flowers.

PER SERVING: ABOUT 248 CAL, 37G PRO, 3G CAR, 9G FAT, 39% CAL FROM FAT, 158MG CHOL, 182MG SOD, 1G FIBER.

Golden Crab Cakes

4 TO 6 SERVINGS

- 8 ounces white beans, cooked*
- 2 tablespoon lemon juice
- ¼ cup canola oil
- 1 pound fresh crabmeat (or sea legs)
- 1 bunch scallions, chopped
- ¼ cup celery, chopped
- 1 teaspoon cumin
- 1 teaspoon paprika
- ½ cup coarse cornmeal
- 2 egg whites
  Nonstick cooking spray
  Lemons, for wedges

In food processor, puree white beans with lemon juice and canola oil. Flake crabmeat and mix well with beans. Add other ingredients and stir gently until well combined. Form into 4 to 6 crab cakes and refrigerate 1 hour.

In a heavy skillet, with nonstick cooking spray, sauté cakes until golden brown. Serve hot with lemon wedges.

PER SERVING: ABOUT 388 CAL, 32G PRO, 29G CAR, 16G FAT, 36% CAL FROM FAT, 101MG CHOL, 417MG SOD, 4G FIBER.

*Note: If canned beans are used, rinse thoroughly to remove as much salt as possible.

© HeartSmart Foods

Spicy Baked Red Snapper Tacos

6 SERVINGS

1   pound red snapper (or grouper) fillets
½   cup fresh cilantro leaves and stems, roughly chopped, divided
3   green onions, finely chopped
1   tablespoon olive oil
¼   cup fresh lime juice
1   teaspoon fresh oregano
2   pounds green tomatillos, husks intact
1   fresh chili pepper, seeded and minced (optional)
12 salt-free corn tortillas, lightly dampened and wrapped in foil
4   cups shredded lettuce

Prepare fire in charcoal grill or preheat oven to 400°.

In a shallow pan, place snapper fillets. Add ¼ cup cilantro, green onions, oil, lime juice, and oregano. Refrigerate 20 minutes.

On a baking tray in oven, place tomatillos. Cook, turning once or twice, about 5 to 8 minutes, or until skins start to bulge. Remove tomatillos from heat and discard husks.

Quarter tomatillos and place in food processor fitted with metal blade. Add the remaining ¼ cup cilantro and chili pepper. Pulse to chop tomatillos. Set aside.

In oven, place package of tortillas. Remove snapper from cilantro mixture; discard marinade. In a shallow roasting pan, place snapper. Cook, turning once, until opaque when pierced with knife, about 4 to 5 minutes on each side. Cut into large chunks.

Remove tortillas from foil. Spoon equal amounts of fish onto each tortilla and top with equal amounts of tomatillo salsa and lettuce.

PER SERVING: About 265 cal, 21g pro, 41g car, 4g fat, 12% cal from fat, 28mg chol, 49mg sod, 8g fiber.

Sautéed Spinach and Leeks

4 SERVINGS

1 tablespoon olive oil
2 leeks, green and white parts, thinly sliced
1 teaspoon fresh lemon juice
1 pound fresh spinach leaves (about 3 bunches), tough stems removed
1/8 teaspoon freshly ground pepper
1 teaspoon finely grated lemon zest
1 teaspoon sherry vinegar

In a heavy saucepan, over medium heat, heat olive oil. Add leeks and sauté 4 to 5 minutes, stirring occasionally, until leeks are softened and translucent. Add lemon juice and spinach leaves. Reduce heat, cover, and cook 4 minutes without removing lid. Uncover and toss to mix well. Add ground pepper, lemon zest, and vinegar and cook, stirring, 1 minute longer. Serve.

PER SERVING: ABOUT 65 CAL, 3G PRO, 7G CAR, 4G FAT, 47% CAL FROM FAT, 0MG CHOL, 70MG SOD, 3G FIBER.

Dannii's Grilled Salmon Tabouli

8 SERVINGS

2 pounds salmon fillet, skinned
6 ounces bulgur (cracked wheat)
Ground black pepper
Juice of 4 limes
4 tablespoons olive oil
1 bunch flat parsley, roughly chopped
6 tablespoons mint, chopped
2 bunches spring onions, finely sliced
6 plum tomatoes, seeded and diced

Char-grill or grill salmon 3 minutes on each side. Set aside to cool. Meanwhile, in a large bowl, soak bulgur in cold water for 10 minutes; drain and squeeze dry. Place bulgur in a bowl and season with black pepper to taste. Add lime juice and olive oil and leave for 30 minutes. While waiting, flake salmon into small pieces.

Add salmon, parsley, mint, and onions to bulgur. Tip into large bowl. Top with plum tomatoes. Cover with food wrap. Drizzle with more olive oil to serve.

PER SERVING: ABOUT 294 CAL, 27G PRO, 23G CAR, 11G FAT, 34% CAL FROM FAT, 59MG CHOL, 91MG SOD, 7G FIBER.

Roasted Corn and Red Pepper Salsa

6 SERVINGS (ABOUT 1 ½ CUPS)

3 ears of fresh corn
1 medium red bell pepper, seeded and quartered
2 tablespoons olive oil, divided
¼ cup lemon juice
1 tablespoon finely chopped parsley
2 garlic cloves, finely chopped
Fresh black pepper to taste

Preheat broiler.

Brush corn and bell pepper lightly with 1 tablespoon olive oil. Broil about 10 minutes, until corn is lightly charred and skin of pepper is blackened and blistered.

Place peppers in plastic food storage bag; close tightly. Let stand 30 minutes, or until skin is loosened. With a small knife, remove skin; chop peppers.

With a large knife, remove kernels from corn. In a medium bowl, combine remaining 1 tablespoon oil, lemon juice, parsley, and garlic.

Cover and refrigerate until serving time. Season with fresh black pepper to taste.

PER SERVING: ABOUT 69 CAL, 1G PRO, 7G CAR, 5G FAT, 58% CAL FROM FAT, 0MG CHOL, 4MG SOD, 1G FIBER.

Raspberry-Nectarine Ice

8 SERVINGS (MAKES 4 CUPS)

5 nectarines, pureed
¾ cup apple juice, white grape juice, or water
1 cup fresh raspberries, pureed

Combine nectarines, juice or water, and berries in a large bowl. Transfer to ice cream maker and prepare according to manufacturer's directions. Thirty minutes before serving, transfer mixture to blender and blend until smooth. Refreeze until serving time.

PER SERVING: ABOUT 56 CAL, 1G PRO, 14G CAR, 1G FAT, 7% CAL FROM FAT, 0MG CHOL, 1MG SOD, 2G FIBER.

Roasted Tomato and Garlic Soup

4 SERVINGS

2 large garlic bulbs
3 tomatoes, chopped and seeded
1 bunch scallions, minced
2 tablespoons chopped fresh parsley
2 cups salt-free chicken or vegetable stock
White pepper to taste
1 teaspoon fresh thyme
2 tablespoons chopped red pepper

Preheat oven to 375°.

Roast whole garlic until soft, about 20 minutes. Remove all skin and crush cloves to a paste. Add to a soup pot with all other ingredients except red pepper and cook on medium heat until tomatoes are soft, about 10 to 15 minutes. Place in blender and mix well. Serve with a sprinkle of chopped red pepper on top.

PER SERVING: ABOUT 70 CAL, 8G PRO, 14G CAR, 2G FAT, 14% CAL FROM FAT, 0MG CHOL, 33MG SOD, 2G FIBER.

© HeartSmart Foods

Spicy Yellow Lentil Stew

8 SERVINGS

1 pound yellow lentils
2 tablespoons olive oil
1 cup onion, chopped
1 cup celery, chopped
½ cup carrots, chopped
½ cup green bell pepper, chopped
½ cup zucchini, sliced
½ cup tomatoes, chopped
5 garlic cloves
1 bay leaf
1 jalapeño pepper, seeded and chopped
½ cup lemon juice
⅛ teaspoon cayenne pepper
2 whole cloves
1 quart salt-free chicken stock

In a large bowl, wash lentils in cold water; set aside.

In large saucepan or Dutch oven, over low heat, heat oil. Sauté onion, celery, carrots, bell pepper, zucchini, tomatoes, garlic, bay leaf, and jalapeño about 5 to 8 minutes, or until tender. Add lemon juice, cayenne pepper, cloves, lentils, and chicken stock. Simmer over medium-low heat for 40 minutes, stirring occasionally.

PER SERVING: ABOUT 262 CAL, 22G PRO, 40G CAR, 5G FAT, 16% CAL FROM FAT, 0MG CHOL, 44MG SOD, 19G FIBER.

Oriental Grilled Chicken

6 SERVINGS

- ¼ cup canola oil
- 4 tablespoons rice vinegar
- 4 tablespoons balsamic vinegar
- 2 tablespoons minced fresh ginger
- 2 tablespoons minced fresh garlic
- ½ Vidalia onion, thinly sliced
- 1 tablespoon spice powder (also known as 5-spice powder)
- 2 pounds chicken breasts, skinned and boned

In a shallow baking dish, mix seven marinade ingredients well. Add chicken breasts and turn to coat each one with marinade. Cover and refrigerate until ready to grill. (Overnight gives chicken the best flavor.) While grilling, brush chicken with marinade. When ready to serve, slice breasts into ½-inch strips.

PER SERVING: ABOUT 257 CAL, 35G PRO, 3G CAR, 11G FAT, 40% CAL FROM FAT, 88MG CHOL, 99MG SOD, 0G FIBER.

© HeartSmart Foods

High Voltage Banana-Strawberry Shake

4 SERVINGS

- 6 cups nonfat milk
- 3 medium bananas, peeled, sliced, frozen
- 1 teaspoon vanilla extract
- 1 teaspoon almond extract
- 1 cup strawberries, sliced
- 1 teaspoon ground cinnamon

In blender container, combine all ingredients except cinnamon. Blend until smooth, about 30 seconds. Pour into glasses. Sprinkle cinnamon on top.

PER SERVING: ABOUT 130 CAL, 9G PRO, 22G CAR, 1G FAT, 5% CAL FROM FAT, 4MG CHOL, 127MG SOD, 1G FIBER.

Roasted Rosemary Lamb

4 SERVINGS

4   loins of lamb (4 ounces each)
⅛   teaspoon black pepper
2   tablespoons chopped fresh rosemary leaves
1   tablespoon grated orange rind
    Nonstick cooking spray
1   cup balsamic vinegar

Remove excess fat from lamb.

In a small bowl combine pepper, rosemary, and orange rind. Sprinkle over lamb loins.

In a medium sauté pan, over medium-high flame, with nonstick cooking spray, sauté lamb to desired doneness. Remove from pan to plate. Deglaze pan with balsamic vinegar and reduce by half. Serve over lamb loins immediately.

PER SERVING: ABOUT 346 CAL, 30G PRO, 4G CAR, 23G FAT, 61% CAL FROM FAT, 112MG CHOL, 89MG SOD, 0G FIBER.

Summer Squash Bisque

6 SERVINGS

    Nonstick cooking spray or 2 to 3 tablespoons canola oil
1   medium onion, chopped
4 to 6 summer squash, sliced
2   cups salt-free chicken stock
4   tablespoons cilantro, chopped
½   cup low-fat sour cream
1   teaspoon ground coriander
½   teaspoon white pepper
    Rice cakes, as accompaniment

In a soup pot, with nonstick cooking spray, sauté onion. When translucent add squash, chicken stock, and cilantro. Simmer 10 to 15 minutes. Transfer to a food processor and puree. Add sour cream, coriander, and white pepper. Blend. Serve with rice cakes.

PER SERVING: ABOUT 111 CAL, 1G PRO, 9G CAR, 8G FAT, 57% CAL FROM FAT, 2MG CHOL, 21MG SOD, 3G FIBER.

© HeartSmart Foods

Dungeon Dungeness Crab Salad

During my frequent visits to the Hamptons, I often stay at the castle of Princes Alan and Ivan Wilzig (of the blood royal, naturally), and am cosseted in the lap of luxury by the castle's majordomo, Steven Welch, who has shared these recipes for Dungeon Dungeness Crab Salad, Tower Tabouli, and Swordfish Salad Niçoise (on page 254) from their private chef, Erik Tyree.

6 SERVINGS

3 pounds Dungeness crab, steamed, shelled, and picked over
2 heads endive, roughly diced
1 cup low-fat yogurt
Juice of ½ lemon
3 cups mesclun salad mix, washed and spun dry

Have your serfs mix the first 4 ingredients and arrange attractively on greens.

PER SERVING: About 252 cal, 44g pro, 11g car, 3g fat, 11% cal from fat, 136mg chol, 735mg sod, 5g fiber.

Tower Tabouli

4 SERVINGS

1 package (12 ounces) salt-free tabouli mix (prepared following package instructions)
4 plum tomatoes, cubed
1 large cucumber, diced
4 green onions, white and green parts, diced
1 cup fresh parsley, minced
¼ cup extra-virgin olive oil
⅛ cup lemon juice

In a large bowl, mix all ingredients and let flavors meld for several hours in refrigerator. Serve chilled.

PER SERVING: About 359 cal, 7g pro, 36g car, 24g fat, 56% cal from fat, 0mg chol, 252mg sod, 6g fiber.

Vegetarian Chili

4 SERVINGS

1 cup onions, chopped
2 cups celery, chopped
2 tomatoes, chopped
2 cups salt-free vegetable stock
1 cup broccoli florets
½ cup zucchini, chopped
8 ounces kidney beans, cooked
2 garlic cloves, minced
3 teaspoons cumin
1 teaspoon cinnamon
Pepper to taste
Sour cream or yogurt, for garnish

In a large pot, on medium heat, cook onions, celery, and tomatoes in vegetable stock until tender, about 10 minutes. Add all other ingredients and simmer on low heat for 30 to 40 minutes. Serve with a dollop of sour cream or yogurt.

PER SERVING: ABOUT 212 CAL, 11G PRO, 39G CAR, 3G FAT, 11% CAL FROM FAT, 1MG CHOL, 68MG SOD, 8G FIBER.

© HeartSmart Foods

Southwestern-Style Turkey Cassoulet

3 TO 4 SERVINGS

1 pound turkey breast
2 tablespoons olive oil
5 garlic cloves
¼ cup apple cider vinegar
½ cup carrots, cubed
½ cup onion, cubed
½ cup tomato, cubed
½ cup okra, cubed
1 cup cooked white beans
⅛ teaspoon cayenne pepper
Pinch nutmeg
⅛ teaspoon black pepper
Fresh thyme to taste

Cut turkey into ½-inch cubes. In large sauté pan, heat oil. Add turkey and brown. Add remaining ingredients. Simmer for 25 minutes on low heat.

PER SERVING: ABOUT 357 CAL, 38G PRO, 16G CAR, 15G FAT, 39% CAL FROM FAT, 84MG CHOL, 88MG SOD, 3G FIBER.

Citrus-Grilled Turkey Salad

4 SERVINGS

1 cup grapefruit juice
1 cup orange juice
½ cup chopped red onion
2 teaspoons jalapeño pepper
⅛ cup honey
1 pound turkey breast cutlets
Mixed greens
2 cups oranges, cut in segments
2 cups pink grapefruit, cut in segments
¼ cup lime juice
4 tomatoes, seeded and diced, for garnish
¼ cup cilantro, for garnish

In a saucepan, bring grapefruit and orange juices, onion, jalapeño pepper, and honey to a boil. Reduce heat. Simmer until liquid is reduced by half. Strain reserve liquid and cool. Pour ⅔ marinade over turkey cutlets, reserving remaining marinade in a bowl for dressing.

Grill marinaded turkey cutlets, 2 minutes on each side.

Arrange turkey cutlets on mixed greens, and slice turkey. Add orange and grapefruit segments.

To marinade, add lime juice. Spoon over cutlets. Garnish with tomatoes and cilantro.

PER SERVING: ABOUT 346 CAL, 26G PRO, 47G CAR, 8G FAT, 20% CAL FROM FAT, 66MG CHOL, 77MG SOD, 5G FIBER.

Onion and Pineapple Salsa

12 SERVINGS

1¼ cups chopped sweet onion
½ cup chopped red bell pepper
½ cup chopped green bell pepper
1½ cups chopped pineapple
3 teaspoons chopped fresh cilantro

In a medium bowl, combine all ingredients. Cover and refrigerate several hours to let flavors blend.

PER SERVING: ABOUT 12 CAL, 0G PRO, 3G CAR, 0G FAT, 0% CAL FROM FAT, 0MG CHOL, 1MG SOD, 1G FIBER.

Tenderloin of Beef L'Orange

6 SERVINGS

2 pounds beef tenderloin, whole
2 tablespoons olive oil
1 tablespoon cracked black pepper
Nonstick cooking spray
4 tablespoons minced onions
½ cup beef stock, unsalted
Juice from 2 large oranges
2 cups broccoli florets
3 cups brown rice, cooked
1 orange, peeled and sliced

Preheat oven to 450°F.

Rub beef with olive oil and black pepper. Roast 10 to 12 minutes, until just done. Meanwhile, in a large skillet, with nonstick cooking spray, sauté onions. When just brown, add beef stock and orange juice. Cook on medium high until sauce begins to thicken. Steam broccoli in vegetable steamer.

To serve, slice beef in ¼-inch pieces; layer on plate with broccoli and rice. Cover beef with sauce and orange slices.

PER SERVING: ABOUT 566 CAL, 32G PRO, 30G CAR, 36G FAT, 57% CAL FROM FAT, 106MG CHOL, 110MG SOD, 4G FIBER.

© HeartSmart Foods

Party Baked
Potato Crisps

4 SERVINGS

2 tablespoons olive oil, divided, or olive oil cooking spray
2 baking potatoes, ½ to ¾ pounds each, unpeeled, scrubbed
Freshly ground black pepper
1 teaspoon chopped fresh chives

Preheat oven to 400°.

Oil two nonstick baking sheets with 1 tablespoon olive oil, or cooking spray. Cut the potatoes into slices ⅛-inch thick. In a medium bowl, place potatoes and toss with remaining tablespoon olive oil to coat evenly, or coat with cooking spray. Season slices with black pepper, and place on prepared baking sheet. Bake 20 to 25 minutes, until crisp and browned. Transfer to serving dish and toss with chives.

PER SERVING: ABOUT 166 CAL, 3G PRO, 24G CAR, 7G FAT, 37% CAL FROM FAT, 0MG CHOL, 8MG SOD, 2G FIBER.

Spicy Potato Chips

6 SERVINGS

Nonstick cooking spray
2 pounds baking potatoes, well scrubbed, unpeeled, and cut into ⅛-inch-thick slices
½ teaspoon freshly ground black pepper
1 garlic clove, peeled and finely minced
1 teaspoon paprika
½ teaspoon cayenne pepper
½ teaspoon coarsely cracked black pepper
1½ teaspoons chopped fresh parsley

Preheat oven to 400°.

Lightly coat 2 nonstick baking sheets with nonstick cooking spray. Place potatoes in a shallow bowl; coat lightly with nonstick cooking spray. Sprinkle with ground black pepper. Arrange potatoes slices in a single layer on baking sheets. Bake until crispy brown, about 20 to 25 minutes.

While potatoes are baking, in a large bowl, stir together garlic, paprika, cayenne pepper, cracked black pepper, and parsley. When potatoes are done, add them to bowl of seasonings; toss gently to coat.

PER SERVING: ABOUT 90 CAL, 2G PRO, 21G CAR, 0G FAT, 0% CAL FROM FAT, 0MG CHOL, 7MG SOD, 2G FIBER.

Acknowledgments

My heartfelt thanks and love to two special members of my extended family. To Dr. Judy Kuriansky (my cosmic sister!), whom I love with all my heart (I wouldn't want to be on this planet without her). Thanks for all your on-target advice and guidance during the writing of this book, and every other aspect of my life. And to Elaine Lewis. You've been everything to me—a dear friend, a mother, a sister, a mentor, and much, much more. I cherish the fact that I truly know you will always be there for me—this is no small statement. I love you.

To other extended family members: To Lynn Butler, my closet "glitter queen" who first helped me create High Voltage, so many years ago. Your creative, insightful, intuitive guidance has been a strong force in my life. Finally, here we go! To Alan Wilzig, Karin Hanssen, and Ivan Wilzig—treasured friends whom I adore with all my heart. I am grateful for everything (especially the most fabulous birthday an Energy Queen could have at your Magical Castle). To my "baby" Vivian Bernell—I couldn't love you more if you were my own daughter. You are always in my heart. To Dana Barker, who has also always been there, to talk to, to run things by, whenever I feel a little disconnected. You are one of *my* personal switches. I love you—you are so talented. To Jimmy Hester—at the end of the day, I always say, you are a genius, truly one of a kind (takes one to know one). I do love you—and thank you so very, very, very, very much. To James Edstrom, who has photographed me from day one. We certainly do have a special bond. Thanks for being around so long. To Jeffrey Gurian, who has been there with me for the whole ride—up and down . . . and up again! To Robert Hantman, who was really there when I needed someone to be there (I will never forget that!). And to Harlan, my talented and creative best buddy. I doubt if I could ever live with anyone again. Your bedroom is still empty! Love ya!

To all the talented doctors and professionals, who are also my friends, who help me keep High Voltage looking *fierce:* Dr. Andrew Ordon—for giving me the best accessories a girl could have—you do great tits! (and many other things, of course). Rob Lucas, the only man who truly causes me pain, but who keeps my lines and lips poufy—thank you very much! Hair stylist Steven Dillon, who keeps my not-so-terrific hair looking fab. Montgomery Frazier, who has done so much more than help me keep my look together all these years (you *are* precious to me!) Mark Bauer—I can always count on you to help me look fabulous (your gowns are gorgeous!). Imir at Deviations—your clothes are fierce! I am so happy I found you guys! Maria Alonso, the best masseuse in the world. All the folks at Mario Badescu for taking such good care of my skin all these years. Dr. B. Marina Torrelio, Emery Castore, and James V. Polito at Better Health Natural Foods—who feed me whenever I'm in town. Without you I would die. And especially to my dear Dr. Neils Lauerson, whose generosity has been beyond belief. Thank you for watching over me all these years (and to Joan, in your office, for always fitting me in).

To all my dedicated advisers and friends who have been of help to me: Jimmy Hester, who literally took me by the hand to Joel Fotinos at Putnam, who took me to John Duff—where the sparks really flew! Joel Fotinos, for getting my message—and acting on it so quickly. John Duff, my brilliant, so handsome, so sophisticated publisher, who is truly my number one Cosmic Commander—thank you, thank you, thank you!

To my literary agent, Lisa Bankoff at ICM, for pulling together all the loose ends; to Joel Weinstein, my attorney, who insisted I read my contract (I was so happy to get it, I didn't care); to ICM's dynamo Jonny Podell, who plays a much bigger part in my life than he knows (or possibly cares), but I love him more than even I understand—time will tell!).

To my darling Alvaro, a true artist in every sense of the word. You have always been so very special to me—your talent is astounding, your drawings are magnificent. I am so looking forward to all the wonderful projects we will be doing together. To all my wonderful chefs—and especially the gorgeous Victor Swainson, whom my clients adore, and who has been a treat to work with. Thanks for all your help in helping to develop recipes that are truly High Voltage! To Jim Jondreau of HeartSmart, for his wonderful healthy recipes, and Steven Welch, majordomo of the castle, and Erik Tyree; thanks to Andi Watstein, for her last-minute work on the nutritional information in the recipes; to Dr. Robin Stern-Mannis, for her energy and for letting me rip apart her kitchens and to Anne Marie Dunatov Purdy, Marion Asnes, and Geoff Bailey for their research and much needed help; to Lisa Arcella, for her efforts on my behalf; to Miles Chavetz, restaurateur, who always puts himself out for me. You are a doll! To my outrageous, one-of-a-kind Peggy Packer—I bow to you (and you know I really do).

To David Granoff, my first publicist, who put me on the map; Richard Rubinstein, Couri Hay, and all the other people who keep me there; and especially, again, Jimmy Hester, Jason Weinberg, and Ed Callahan, who are gonna help me put this book on the map—what a crew, if I say so myself. And to my invaluable Richard Valvo—you are one of the most talented and creative people I have ever worked with. I am truly blessed to have you on my team!

Speaking of teams, my thanks to the talented and enthusiastic team at Putnam, who helped make this book and my dream (I dream VERY BIG!) a reality: John, my publisher; my editor, Sheila Curry (boy, did I get lucky—what a pro!)—for her direction and input, thank you, thank you, Sheila!; Marilyn Ducksworth, PR maven, who has almost as much energy as I do, and her fabulous crew, Mih-Ho Cha and Matthew Snyder. I was much more relaxed after meeting all of you. And to all the art directors, designers, copy editors, and staff at Putnam who worked so hard, including Lisa Amoroso, Charles Björklund, Ann Spinelli, Claire Vaccaro, and all the people whom I don't know but who made my book happen. Thank you, all! I hit the jackpot.

To all my press buddies, who help keep the High Voltage switch turned on, especially Richard Johnson of the *New York Post*'s Page Six, who first recognized that I was an energy conductor; George Rush and Joanna Molloy of the *Daily News,* who have always treated me fairly; *New York* magazine's Ariel Kaminer; plus Neal Travis, Cindy Adams, Michael Musto, A. J. Benza, Nora Lowlar, my supporters at *Vogue, Harper's Bazaar, Elle, New York* magazine, *Town & Country,* and all the other glamorous mags—thanks! And to all the talented photographers who have kept me in the public eye—James Edstrom, Patrick McMullen, Richard Corkery, Aubrey Reuben, Bill Cunningham, Rose Hartman, Diane Cohen, David Allan, Ron Galella, Julie Bernstein, Albert Ferreria, and all the others (you know who you are!). Thank you! I hope it's gonna get easier to place my photos, after this.

To the posse at KTU: head honcho and program director Frankie Blue, music director Andy Shane, and all-around cutie pie Jeff Z., morning show producer Joey B., Kevin Vislocky, who cleans up my radio spots, and my dear buddy Freddy Colon. And to Michelle Visage, a walking, talking, high-energy inspiration, who has truly taken the High Voltage lifestyle and made it her own; I am so proud of her! Thanks to all of you for your support.

And of course, to the one and only Queen of All Media, my good, good buddy and sweetie, RuPaul: Your love and support mean so much to me. I am truly honored to be part of *your* support team. It's one of my top personal missions to always help you keep *your* energy up—so many people love and depend on you. You mean so much to so many (including me!). And to your precious George, whom I love very much—he's my favorite dancing partner.

To Glenn Fricia, my music director and wizard with "the mix"—I've been looking for someone like you for a long time. We make quite a team! And thank you, Andy Giancola, for making Glenn eat . . .

And finally, my love and thanks to all my fabulous clients, who happen to be my dear friends. I can't mention all of you here, but I know you may see yourselves in this book! Special thanks go to David Blaine, Downtown Julie Brown, Jay Cashman, Maria Christiansen, Taylor Dayne, Nancy Davis, Lisa Gilford, Jane Holzer, Tama Janowitz, Beverly Johnson, John King, Laura King, Beverly Peele, Billy Porter, Daniella Rich, and Rick Wake.

To my dear client and best buddy Dannii Minogue, whom I have watched transform into one of my truly fiercest bodies. We've been through so much together; I know I've put you through a few "unusual" situations and I thank you so much for always being there for me. Thank God you have a sense of humor!

My most heartfelt appreciation and love to a very special person, Denise Rich, a terrific client and friend, who gives so much with an open hand and heart, and who has made many things possible for me. Your energy is truly unique! Thank you for everything, including so generously lending me your Hampton home, whenever I needed it, and where so much of this book was written, rewritten, and polished with the help of Allison Kyle Leopold, my creative, articulate, extremely pretty (she hates when I say that!), and very patient co-writer. The "write" collaborator makes all the difference. Energy Up! Whoo!

—HIGH VOLTAGE, 1997

Bibliography

Hampe, Edward C., Jr., and Merle Wittenberg, *The Lifeline of America: The Development of the Food Industry* (New York: McGraw-Hill, 1964).

Heifetz, Jeanne, *Green Groceries: A Mail Order Guide to Organic Foods* (New York: Harper Perennial, 1992).

Heller, Dr. Rachael F., and Dr. Richard F. Heller, *The Carbohydrate Addict's Diet: The Lifelong Solution to Yo-yo Dieting.* (New York: Signet Books, 1991).

Natow, Annette B., Ph.D., R. D., and Jo Ann Heslin, M.A., R.D., *The Supermarket Nutrition Counter* (New York: Pocket Books, 1997).

Nutrition Action Healthletter (Washington DC: Center for Science in the Public Interest). (1875 Connecticut Avenue NW, Suite 300, Washington, DC 20009.)

Peale, Norman Vincent, *The Power of Positive Thinking* (New York: Prentice-Hall, 1952).

Sears, Barry, Ph.D., with Bill Lawren, *The Zone* (New York: Reganbooks/HarperCollins, 1995).

Sheppard, Kay, *Food Addiction: The Body Knows* (Deerfield Park, FL: Health Communications, 1989).

Shinn, Florence Scovel, *The Complete Writings of Florence Scovel Shinn* (Del Rey, CA: DeVorss, 1997).

University of California at Berkeley Wellness Letter, *The New Wellness Encyclopedia of Food and Nutrition* (Somerville, MA: Houghton Mifflin, 1995).

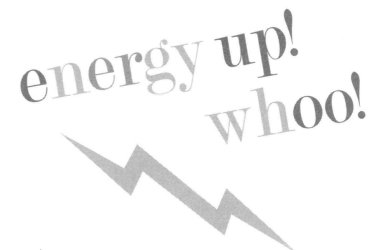